Frankenfoods —

Controversy, Lies and Health Risks

Frankenfoods —

Controversy, Lies and Health Risks

Michael B. Wald, MD, DC, MS, CNS, CCN, CDN

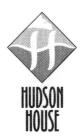

HUDSON
HOUSE

These materials are meant for educational purposes only and are not to substitute for independent research or medical advice.

ISBN: 978-1-58776-956-6

Disclaimer
The information, concepts and ideas in this book are ever evolving and may change over the course of time. The author of this book has presented this information for educational purposes only. This information should not be used as medical or health advice, nor to substitute for sound nutritional advice.

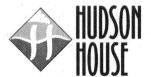

HUDSON
HOUSE

675 Dutchess Turnpike, Poughkeepsie, NY 12603
www.hudsonhousepub.com   (800) 724-1100

TABLE OF CONTENTS

FOREWORD

Dr. Michael Wald, author of **Frankenfoods - Controversy, Lies & Your Health**, offers a riveting perspective of the GMO predicament, exploring governmental and industry cover-ups, health dangers, environmental threats, GMO-free food plans and recipes, nutritional supplements and other practical solutions. Dr. Wald declares, "*The GMO dilemma is here to stay. Anyone interested in protecting their health and that of their loved ones, friends and the planet must educate themselves and take political and personal action right now!*"

ACKNOWLEDGEMENTS

This book has been a necessary step in my own education and inquiry into the GMO controversy. I must acknowledge each and every one of my readers for taking the time and effort to improve your life, the lives of others and the health of our precious planet by exploring how GMOs impact your health now and will continue to far into the future.

I would like to thank my family, including my wife, Robin; my sons, Aaron and Eli; and especially my daughter, Maya, who carried out much of the research that made this book possible. I am blessed to have my beautiful daughter, Maya, in my life and am awed by her fortitude and sharp mind and for motivating me to be my best. To my wife, Robin, I am grateful for her intelligence and ability to see into the hearts of people. To my eldest son, Aaron, for finding what he loves in life, working harder than anyone for it and for challenging me. And to Eli, my youngest son, for his extreme and special creativity and for allowing me to share in his profound way of experiencing and expressing life.

The Complimentary/Alternative Medicine (CAM) community, of which I consider myself and my works a part, deserves special mention for the passion, dedication and intelligent perspective healers in this community apply to natural health. The CAM industry begins with a fundamental assumption: "If it ain't natural, it's probably bad for you." This simple assumption has proven correct for countless concepts, products and procedures that have been forwarded by the pharmaceutical, industrial and medical complex and promoted for human health, but instead promote disease and loss of quality and length of life. Gluten dangers, the refining and processing of foods, and the use of medications for unnecessary medical procedures, and the widespread use of medications that mask symptoms rather than exploring natural healing options are just a few examples of deleterious practices that are now, more than ever, being challenged by the ever-increasingly intelligent and more health-minded population. The insidious incorporation of GMOs into our lives over the last few decades is among the more recent examples of factors that will increase human suffering and that of other mammals, insects and the planet as a whole.

I would like to extend my thanks to my hard-working and dedicated colleagues, including Nilay Shah, MD; Sunny Seward, CNS; Muhummad Khan, MD; Mark Leder, DC; Daniel Bies, DC; Glen Brady, MD; Jeffrey Bland, PhD; Adam Banning; Jack Kessinger, DC; Virginia Kessenger, DC; the late Winna Henry; my associates and colleagues involved with the International & American Association of Clinical Nutritionists (IAACN); the Chiropractic Board of Clinical Nutrition; the American Chiropractic Association Board of Clinical Nutrition; and the chiropractic profession as a whole.

Finally, I must give special thanks to my father and mother for encouraging me to go for my dreams. To my mother, Sydney, I attribute my creativity and imagination that has forwarded my "out of the box" mindset and has enabled me to help thousands of people during my 25 year career as a leader in the natural health care movement. To my father, Dr. George J. Wald, a chiropractor and nutritionist, I acknowledge his love for chiropractic and nutrition and for cultivating my love of health and wellness early on as a young boy. He would say to me, "It is what is in your heart and head that counts — persevere." My earliest memory of him saying this to me was when I was around the age of three as I lie on his chest looking up at him. My parents' combined support has made me who I am today...and I am grateful!

I will always persevere for the good of my family, my patients, for the world community and for the planet. Thank you all.

Warmly,
Michael Wald

Table of Terms, Acronyms and Abbreviations

ASD (Autism Spectrum Disorders): ASDs are a group of related brain-based disorders that affect a child's behavior, communication and social skills. These disorders include autistic disorder, Asperger syndrome and pervasive developmental disorder-not otherwise specified (PDD-NOS). They are defined by the number and severity of the symptoms.

Autoimmune Disease: This large group of health problems and specific disease states results when our immune system reacts against various cells, tissues and organs as if they were foreign substances. In autoimmune disease, the immune system destroys various body tissues, depending upon the specific type of autoimmune disease, resulting in the symptoms characteristic of the disease. Autoimmune disease may have a genetic component and is influenced by environmental toxins, stress and other exposures.

Beta Toxins: These toxins are produced by various bacteria and come in different forms of enzymes that are toxic to a variety of cells in the body, including fibroblasts, erythrocytes, leukocytes, and macrophages. In terms of insects, Beta toxins and Beta-exotoxins contribute to the internal toxicity of an insect when consumed.

Biolistic Method: A biolistic particle delivery system, or "gene gun," originally designed for plant transformation, is a device for injecting cells with genetic information. The payload is an elemental particle of a heavy metal coated with plasmid DNA. This technique is often simply referred to as *bioballistics* or *biolistics*. This device is able to transform almost any type of cell, including plants.

BT (Bacillus Thuringiensis): BT is a soil-dwelling bacteria used as a biological chemical pesticide. Found naturally in the stomachs of caterpillars, butterflies and moths and elsewhere in nature, it is considered by the biotech industry to be a natural pesticide.

Bt Corn: This corn has been genetically modified to express the Cry1Ab protein of *Bacillus thuringiensis* to kill lepidopteran pests.

Bt Seed: These seeds have been genetically manufactured to produce, in the final crop of corn, the Cry1ab protein *Bacillus thuringiensis* (Bt) to kill lepidopteran pests.

CCD (Colony Collapse Disorder): CCD refers to a phenomenon effecting worker bees of the European honeybee whose colonies abruptly disappear. Many agricultural crops worldwide are pollinated by bees; their disappearance results in serious economic and environmental impacts.

CDC (Center of Disease Control): A U.S. federal agency established to help safeguard public health by control and prevention of disease, disability and injury in the U.S., the CDC is headquartered in Atlanta, GA. Its main focus is on infectious disease, environmental health, food-borne pathogens, health promotion, injury prevention and occupational safety and health.

Chromosome: Found in cells, a chromosome is an organized structure of DNA, protein and RNA. It is a single piece of coiled DNA containing many genes, regulatory elements and other nucleotide sequences. Chromosomes also contain DNA-bound proteins, which serve to package the DNA and control its functions. Chromosomal DNA encodes most or all of an organism's genetic information; some species also contain plasmids or other extrachromosomal genetic elements.

DDT (Dichlorodiphenyltrichloroethane): DDT is an odorless and tasteless organochlorine compound with insecticidal properties produced by the chemical manufacturer Monsanto. First used to control typhus and malaria during the second half of World War II, DDT was eventually indiscriminately sprayed throughout the U.S., contributing to ongoing acute and chronic health effects, including various cancers, in both humans and wildlife. Its effects often damage our genetic material (DNA), creating birth defects through successive generations.

Desired Traits: Geneticists can often select certain beneficial or *desired* traits by gene manipulation, expressing in genes so that the organism displays those traits. Natural selection favors those genes that best suit the environment.

Detoxification: This is a process whereby body organs, primarily the liver and kidneys, remove various substances — toxins — produced either within the body or are absorbed into the body from the air, water, food, physical contact or other form of exposure.

DNA (Deoxyribonucleic Acid): DNA is a molecule that encodes the genetic instructions used in the development and functioning of all known living organisms and many viruses. DNA is a nucleic acid; alongside proteins and carbohydrates, nucleic acids compose the three major macromolecules essential for all known forms of life.

Down-regulating Genes: Regulation of gene expression includes a wide range of mechanisms that are used by cells to increase or decrease the production of specific gene products (protein or RNA), and is informally termed *gene regulation*. Down-regulation is a term referring to reducing the amount of certain products produced as a result of gene expression.

EPA (Environmental Protection Agency): The EPA is a U.S. federal agency originally created by former president Richard Nixon to protect human health and the environment by establishing and reinforcing laws passed by congress.

Equivalency: Equivalency suggests that the final traits and inherent quality of the organism produced through the process of genetic manipulation are substantially equivalent, or nearly identical in composition, to the naturally produced organism.

Farm-grown: There are two types of farm-grown foods: those using the standard farm-industry cultivation techniques such as plows, pesticides, fungicides and herbicides, and those grown organically without the direct use of pesticides, fungicides and herbicides.

FDA (Food and Drug Administration): The FDA is a U.S. federal agency responsible for protecting the public health by assuring the safety, efficacy and security of human and veterinary drugs, biological products, medical devices, our nation's food supply, cosmetics and products that emit radiation. The FDA is also responsible for advancing the public health by helping to speed innovations that make medicines more effective, safer and affordable, and by helping the public get the accurate, science-based information they need to use the appropriate medicines and foods to maintain and improve their health. The FDA also has responsibility for regulating the manufacturing, marketing and distribution of tobacco products to protect the public health and to reduce tobacco use by minors.

FDCA (Federal Food, Drug, and Cosmetic Act): The FDCA (aka FFDCA or FD&C) is a set of laws passed by the U.S. Congress in 1938 giving authority to the FDA to oversee the safety of food, drugs and cosmetics.

Gene Gun: A gene gun, or biolistic particle delivery system, originally designed for plant transformation, is a device for injecting cells with genetic information. The payload is an elemental particle of a heavy metal coated with plasmid DNA. This technique is often simply referred to as *bioballistics* or *biolistics*. This device is able to transform almost any type of cell, including plants.

GMO (Genetically Modified Organism or Food): GMOs are among the most popular terms used to describe foods produced by seeds that have been genetically modified in a laboratory.

Hyperinsulinemia: In this condition, the pancreas, a hormone-secreting and digestive organ, produces and releases excessive amounts of insulin, causing low blood sugar and other health problems.

IGF1 (Insulin-like growth factor, aka somatomedian C): IGF1 is a protein in humans with a similar chemical structure to insulin, another human hormone. In mammals it plays a major role in childhood growth and repair of tissue.

Malabsorption Syndromes: These specific conditions and health problems involve inadequate absorption or malabsorption of various nutrients from foods, including aging and Celiac Disease. People of any age can suffer from malabsorption syndromes, contributing to a large variety of symptoms and diseases.

Natural Selection: Natural selection is the gradual process by which biological traits become either more or less common in a population as a function of the effect of inherited traits on the differential reproductive success of organisms interacting with their environment. It is a key mechanism of evolution. The term "natural selection" was popularized by Charles Darwin, who intended it to be compared to artificial selection, which is now called *selective breeding*.

PCBs (Polychlorinated Biphenyls): This organic pollutant was widely used in capacitors, electric motors, coolant fluids and transformers. Strongly environmentally toxic, PCB production was banned by the U.S. Congress in 1979. This chemical causes various cancers in animals and other mammals.

PCR (Polymerase Chain Reaction): PCR is a technique for amplifying DNA sequences in vitro by separating the DNA into two strands and incubating them with oligonucleotide primers and DNA polymerase. PCR can amplify a specific sequence of DNA by as many as one billion times and is important in biotechnology, forensics, medicine and genetic research.

Pesticides: A pesticide is generally a chemical or biological agent (such as a virus, bacterium, antimicrobial or disinfectant) that through its effect deters, incapacitates, kills or otherwise discourages pests such as insects, plant pathogens, weeds, mollusks, birds, mammals, fish, nematodes (roundworms) and microbes that destroy property, cause nuisance, spread disease or are vectors for disease. The most common use of pesticides is as *plant protection products* (also known as *crop protection products*), which in general protect plants from damaging influences such as weeds, diseases or insects. This use of pesticides is so common that the term *pesticide* is often treated as synonymous with plant protection product, although it is in fact a broader term, as pesticides are also used for non-agricultural purposes. Although there are benefits to the use of pesticides, some also have drawbacks, such as potential toxicity to humans and other animals. According to the Stockholm Convention on Persistent Organic Pollutants, nine of the twelve most dangerous and persistent organic chemicals are pesticides.

Phenylalanine: Found naturally in the breast milk of mammals, phenylalanine is used in the manufacture of food and drink products and sold as a nutritional supplement for its reputed analgesic and antidepressant effects. It is a direct precursor to the neuromodulator phenylethylamine, a commonly used dietary supplement.

PIP (Plant-Incorporated Protectants): PIPs are pesticidal substances produced by plants and the genetic material necessary for the plant to produce the substance. For example, scientists can take the gene for a specific Bt pesticidal protein and introduce the gene into the plant's genetic material. Then the plant manufactures the pesticidal protein that controls the pest when it feeds on the plant. Both the protein and its genetic material are regulated by the EPA; the plant itself is not regulated.

rGBH (bovine somatotropin or somatotrophin): Produced by the pituitary gland of a cow, this peptide (protein) hormone regulates various metabolic processes. Genentech, a biotech company, discovered and patented the gene in the 1970s. Various biotech companies, including Monsanto, developed commercial rBST products that were eventually approved by the U.S. Food and Drug Administration.

RNA (Ribonucleic Acid): This large protein molecule plays a vital role in the genetic coding, decoding, regulation and expression of genes. RNA, along with another vital genetic biological molecule known as DNA, comprises large molecules (macromolecules) fundamentally essential for the formation and perpetuation of life.

Roundup® Ready Crops: Roundup® is Monsanto's trade name for glyphosate (*N*-(phosphonomethyl) glycine), a broad-spectrum systemic herbicide used to kill weeds, especially annual broadleaf weeds and grasses known to compete with commercial crops grown around the globe. Glyphosate was discovered to be an herbicide by Monsanto chemist John E. Franz in 1970. Monsanto brought it to market in the 1970s; their last commercially relevant U.S. patent expired in 2000.

Superweeds: These weeds have developed a tolerance to the broad-spectrum herbicide glyphosate.

Toxins: A toxin is a poisonous substance produced within living cells or organisms; synthetic substances created by artificial processes are thus excluded. Toxins can be small molecules, peptides or proteins that are capable of causing disease on contact with or absorption by body tissues interacting with biological macromolecules such as enzymes or cellular receptors. Toxins vary greatly in their severity, ranging from minor and severe to almost immediately deadly, as in botulinum toxin. *(excerpted from Wikipedia)*

Transfer Vector: When geneticists use small pieces of DNA to clone a gene and create a GMO, that DNA is called a *vector*. The vector serves as the carrier for the transfer or insertion of genes.

Transformation: In molecular biology, transformation is the genetic alteration of a cell resulting from the direct uptake, incorporation and expression of exogenous genetic material (exogenous DNA) from its surroundings and taken up through the cell membrane(s). Transformation occurs naturally in some species of bacteria, but it can also be affected by artificial means in other cells.

Transgenic Plants: These plants are produced from genetically modified seeds.

Wild-type: These plants grow naturally in the wild and have a nutritional content that is dozens to thousands of times higher than farm-grown plants.

Introduction

Frankenfoods — Controversy, Lies and Health Risks is my first organized attempt to answer many questions the public, my patient population and I share regarding the potential health risks, environmental impacts and political implications of introducing genetically modified organisms (GMO) or foods (GMF) into our environment and our bodies. Throughout this book the terms "GMO" and "Frankenfoods" will refer to all genetically modified foods.

As a natural health care provider for nearly 25 years, I have treated patients, educated the public, attended scientific symposia and researched hundreds of topics that involve staying healthy, delaying the onset of disease and improving overall quality of life for people. I predict that the GMO controversy will continue for many years, making it necessary for each of us to become educated on this issue so that we can decide our stance on GMOs and what we should eat. From a human health perspective, I fear that the quality and length of life for people who consume toxic GMOs will be adversely affected. My research has convinced me that some people will endure vague and fleeting symptoms with no obvious cause, and ultimately, over years and even decades, will suffer from severe health issues such as cancer, intestinal problems, fertility issues, fatigue, memory problems and other health disturbances as a direct result of consuming GMOs. Doctors and scientific researchers will attempt to treat these symptoms with other toxic compounds...namely pharmaceutical drugs (some of which contain GMO ingredients)...thus continuing the cycle of symptom suppression and disease in exchange for medication side effects, even though natural solutions are often readily available. As a population we are being force fed foods that have been manipulated unnaturally in a laboratory and are presumed to be safe for human consumption with no scientific evidence of their short- or long-term safety.

Genetic modification of our food supply has the potential to cause devastating health risks. Some of the ways in which GMOs may cause illness and chronic disease include:

- Ingestion of foods our bodies have not adapted to because of their recent introduction into the human food chain
- Indirect health risks and serious environmental impacts, as cross-contamination between GMOs and unintended plants and animals in the surrounding and distant environment can and have already occurred
- Increased cancers and various autoimmune diseases such as Alzheimer's disease, Multiple Sclerosis and Lupus; inflammatory bowel diseases such as Crohn's Disease and ulcerative colitis; and hormonal problems stemming from effects upon our DNA (genetic material) and immune system

Nutritional content is dozens to thousands of times lower in farm-grown crops as opposed to the wild-type food counterparts. GMOs are all farm-grown and therefore are significantly inferior to non-GMO wild-type plants. GMOs, as I have described throughout this book, are more nutrient deficient compared to the wild-type organic plants, carry potentially greater toxins and allergens and may promote antibiotic resistance – and these health impacts are just the "tip of the iceberg."

Dangers to our health from GMO consumption simply cannot be ruled out at this time, and in fact, reasonable scientific evidence and real-life experiences suggest right now that GMOs can and do pose potentially serious health risks. Some health issues will be obvious, but most will be hidden from view in the short-term only to manifest as familiar symptoms and diseases. Most will likely go unrecognized by conventional physicians and the scientific community as resulting from a lifetime of GMO consumption.

Frankenfoods — Controversy, Lies and Health Risks is not a complete review of GMOs, but it is the only book I know of that breaks down many of the important health, political and environmental issues in a question and answer format. Many good books on GMOs are available, but mine is the only source of GMO education that suggests natural ways, in terms of foods and nutritional supplements, to deal with our inevitable exposure to GMOs. Please see a list of suggested reading material at the end of this book. Read as much as you can on this topic if you desire to become better educated, develop a balanced and rational perspective on the GMO issue and become a part of the solution. Sadly, many of my patients, family members, friends and even complete strangers with whom I have spoken about the GMO controversy have little or no knowledge of this issue...an issue that not only will impact them personally and their loved ones and friends, but may pose health risks to all future generations.

The controversy is essentially this: Various governments, government organizations (e.g., the Food and Drug Administration (FDA), the Environmental Protection Agency (EPA), GMO scientists and manufacturers of GMO seeds (e.g., Monsanto) ignored and deny the potential dangers to the world environment and human health solely for profit. Have there been cover-ups? Are we victims of false-science? *Frankenfoods — Controversy, Lies and Health Risks* covers many fundamentals you must know to protect your health, your family's health and the environment in which you live. I believe that we have all been victims of deceit and misrepresentations regarding the safety and environmental impacts of GMOs, and throughout this book I provide many examples of how this has occurred. I am convinced that cover-ups abound and continue to poison us from many influences, including the industrial complex, scientific circles and within the political arena.

Has appropriate scientific study proved beyond reasonable doubt that GMOs are safe for human consumption and the environment? I say *no*. Rigorous and unbiased scientific study is lacking, and the limited study to date supports the concept that GMOs should not have been introduced into our food supply. To paraphrase a geneticist on this topic, one who doubts the uncertainty of the impact of GMOs upon human health and the environment must be either ignorant or plain stupid!

Do GMOs pose strong health risks that overwhelm the potential benefits of GMOs? Has it been established that GMOs are safe in the short- and long-term for human consumption? Have political and financial motivations corrupted and blinded organizations such as the FDA, manufacturers of GMO seeds, the White House and other influential parties to the human health risks? Are these same organizations that we are supposed to trust to police industry for health and safety violations themselves guilty, either directly or indirectly, for slowly poisoning our bodies and our environment, condemning future generations to unprecedented disease and disability?

Frankenfoods — Controversy, Lies and Health Risks will help guide you towards a clearer and more insightful understanding of the current issues involving GMOs. By reading this book you have taken an essential step towards enlightening yourself, but whether you take additional action or not, the GMO controversy is here to stay. You most likely have already been adversely affected by it. GMOs can steal your health, like a parasite that has crept its way into your food, body and environment, in subtle and substantial ways over the course of your life...and will continue to do so unless eliminated.

I have helped my patients through many health problems that stem from various environmental exposures such as chemicals sprayed on our foods, heavy metal contamination, gluten malabsorption, food allergies, food-borne infections, unnaturally processed and denatured food. These food horrors have a super-additive effect, stealing our quality and length of life. I believe these health threats pale in comparison to the risk of GMO consumption.

We have been unwittingly exposed to the most pervasive food and nutritional influence upon our health that has ever existed. But all is not lost. Arm yourself with information and you will develop the resources essential to reverse this dangerous situation we are all being forced to deal with now...namely, the introduction and uncertainty of GMOs.

What Is a Frankenfood?

Remember the book *Frankenstein*, written by Mary Shelley, about a budding young scientist named Frankenstein? Dr. Frankenstein wished to create the perfect, most exquisite human being that ever existed. Instead, young Frankenstein created a ghastly, awful, abhorrent monster. Dr. Frankenstein never imagined that his attempts at improving the human being would result in a literal catastrophe of science and philosophy. Frankenstein mixed his chemicals with various cadaver body parts exactly as he should, certain that he had anticipated every conceivable mishap, but nonetheless he created something completely unlike his desired effect: he produced an abomination — much like the results of the efforts of GMO manufacturers and geneticists.

Frankenfood is a term I chose to describe GMOs to emphasize the Frankenstein-like effects that I believe GMOs are inflicting on our health, society and the planet. GMO scientists imagine, like Dr. Frankenstein, that they can outthink nature's intelligence and improve on nature's evolutionary efforts by creating better foods through unnatural, artificial genetic processes. GMOs are not what they are proposed to be by genetic seed producers like Monsanto that position themselves as sustainable agriculture companies. Many scientific studies to date show unforeseen health problems in humans, other mammals and plants, and to the environment: toxic, allergic, immunologic, cardiac, intestinal, renal, hepatic and other negative health effects that result directly from the consumption of GMOs. However, science should not be the only criteria used to make sound decisions affecting one's health or environment. Public consensus should always be a part of making decisions that affect the one and the many.

Dr. Frankenstein had a misguided but noble purpose when he conceived of creating a more perfect human being. The GMO industry may or may not have some noble purpose behind their efforts to control the source of all food on this planet: *seeds*. It seems, however, based on readily available studies and industry papers about the GMO controversy, the GMO experiment is currently a disastrous failure. Like Frankenstein's monster was to Dr. Frankenstein, GMOs may well be the death of us.

Genetically modified foods include corn and soy products, cottonseed, canola oil, papaya, alfalfa, sugar beets, aspartame and milk. This list is destined to grow unless properly regulated. GMOs are foods produced from seeds that have been artificially modified by geneticists in a laboratory. A gene gun is used to blast desired genes, which carry the potential for certain genetic traits, into the genes of seeds such as corn or soy. The goal of GMO geneticists is to manipulate "normal" or non-GMO food seeds to produce superior foods. Admittedly a tempting concept, but as nature and science would have it, there is a deceitful side to the creation of these "superior" foods — these Frankenfoods.

GMO scientists claim genetic modification will increase food crop yields and thus reduce world hunger and food costs, and improve the nutritional quality of our current food supply. They make other questionable and unsubstantiated claims as well. Sadly, current research, albeit limited and inconclusive for the most part, still suggests that GMOs have inferior nutritional quality, GMO crops yields are not greater and world hunger will not be reduced by GMO technology. We currently produce an average of 4.5 pounds of food per person per day on the planet; the real problem is getting the food to the mouths of people in need.

Frankenfoods represent what can happen, and what is already happening, when mankind attempts to reinvent the "blade of grass." Nature, in all of its brilliance, offers wondrous beauties that we often take for granted — from the skies, oceans, rivers and lakes to the animals and plants, including the grains, fruits and vegetables that help sustain us. Contrary to GMO geneticists' claims, GMOs are not naturally produced and never can be as pro-GMO geneticists would have us believe. Shooting strawberry genes into salmon or tomatoes with gene guns is not a natural genetic change!

Adaptation is a term used by biologists to describe the process whereby living organisms, like you and me and our ancestors, cope with changes in our external environments and internal physiologies. For example, if our human ancestors lived in a cold environment, those early hominids having genetically superior cold weather tolerance would live, procreate and pass on that trait, while those lacking that trait would die off and not pass on their inferior genetic traits. Anthropologists, scientists who study evolution, believe that human beings, as well as other animals and plants, have evolved in this similar manner of continuous adaptation to their environments since the first documented genetic human, *Homo habilis,* evolved around 2.3 million years ago. The fundamental process of genetic evolution has been "reinvented" by modern-day geneticists, and when applied to Frankenfoods, I predict the results will be disastrous.

Domestication of plants has been occurring for over 10,000 years, and has resulted in a certain homeostasis and natural perfection. Nature has designed the evolutionary process to allow for natural development of organisms that match, and keep pace, with spontaneous and gradual genetic alterations in their genes as well as environmental influences. It is simply impossible for the type of gene manipulation induced by geneticists in a laboratory to match nature's perfection. I am not claiming that there is no benefit in society for genetic manipulation of foods; what I am saying is that GMOs should be considered unsafe until thoroughly proven otherwise.

It is difficult, if not impossible, to improve upon nature. Scientific advancement, in particular genetic modification of foods, may have a place in our lives given the right context, and once rigorous human safety and environmental impact studies have been conducted. At this point in time, however, it simply cannot be claimed that GMOs, as a whole, are safe for our bodies or our planet. Scientific evolution and progress always involves setbacks and controversies. What is occurring in the political, economic, agricultural and health sectors will inevitably shift our perception of the world and our health...I fear for the worse.

Questions and Answers

In a time of universal deceit, telling the truth is a revolutionary act.
George Orwell

Questioning is an essential part of our lives. Learning is impossible and progress halted when one does not internalize our observations of the world and form new perceptions of what it all means in our lives. Ignorance grows, scientific progress is halted and personal growth is stifled if we do not constantly question ourselves and the happenings in the world surrounding us. The GMO dilemma has occurred, at least in part I believe, due to a failure of the "powers that be" to ask the right questions. There exists an immaturity of knowledge about GMO safety, because our interconnectedness with our environment has been ignored or is entirely unrecognized by those who support the GMO agenda. The unwavering desire of GMO seed manufacturers to pursue fulfillment of their selfish agendas has created our current environment of societal fear, political corruption and impending health crisis. We cannot exist without the world, but the world can and will exist long after human beings are gone. Why is Monsanto so seemingly convinced that Frankenfoods are safe? I believe that their position on this matter is entirely born out of denial.

This book is my attempt to help "wake up" those scientists, politicians and citizens who have given little thought to or ignored the wellbeing of their fellow man for the sake of financial profit...at the expense of our quality and length of life and our inalienable human rights. When GMOs are involved, the freedom to live lives that we love involves, at least in part, our right to ask questions and consider the answers as they potentially impact our lives, our loved ones and everyone on the planet.

Albert Einstein said, "The important thing is not to stop questioning. Curiosity has its own reason for existing. One cannot help but be in awe when he contemplates the mysteries of eternity, of life, of the marvelous structure of reality. It is enough if one tries merely to comprehend a little of this mystery every day. Never lose a holy curiosity." It is my hope that we all continue to ask questions and maintain an open mind regarding the GMO controversies that we are currently forced to confront. The questions and answers that I have provided in this book are only a starting point for your deep consideration, thoughtfulness and good intentions. To maintain an open mind to both sides of any issue brings with it the ability to consider new options and see things transparently and without bias. When considering the many nuances involved with GMOs and their political, social, moral, financial and health impacts, one realizes that only our educated choices and actions taken can reverse the GMO juggernaut that will otherwise continue unchallenged. Choice is the act of making a decision when given at least two or more options – the GMO industry should not be allowed to make the choice of forcing Frankenfoods into your life without serious opposition.

Choose health!

1. WHAT ARE GENETICALLY MODIFIED ORGANISMS?

The term "genetically modified organism" (GMO) refers to an organism whose genetic material has been modified due to genetic engineering techniques. Genetic modification technologies are used to alter the makeup of organisms such as animals, plants and bacteria. GMOs are the source of many modified foods and are used widely in scientific research to produce other goods as well. In 2006, eight countries grew 97% of the global crops with artificially modified genes: the United States (53%), Argentina (17%), Brazil (11%), Canada (6%), India (4%), China (3%), Paraguay (2%) and South Africa (1%). Within the next decade researchers expect to see a dramatic increase in the use of GMOs and GM technologies in industrialized nations.

Corn Is a Pesticide Factory

Genetically modified organisms such as corn produce their own pesticides. Each ear of corn is literally a "drug manufacturing plant"! Proponents of GMOs frequently claim that current methods used to genetically modify foods are identical to, or not substantially different from, the method naturally occurring in the environment without human intervention. I will venture to say you will never find corn naturally farmed or grown in the wild that has the ability to produce a toxic pesticide all by itself!

Gene Gun

One of the most common methods used to insert genes into a target genetic material or DNA (e.g., corn or soy) is the biolistic method. This method involves using a gene gun to shoot into the target's DNA source a gene or two that carry the desired trait. However, unexpected results from this method may occur including, but not limited to, disrupting the entire genetic sequence of the target, up-regulating genes, down-regulating genes, causing genes to be silent and other unpredictable or undesired effects. These effects are referred to by geneticists as "default effects."

One theoretically possible default effect of this "transgenic gene manipulation" is cancer. Cancer, in part, results in the inappropriate up-regulation of genes known as

11

oncogenes (cancer genes). The changes in the genetic sequence of the target (i.e., seeds) may theoretically result in allergies to new proteins, to gene products or to the original source of the gene or genes (e.g., peanuts) being blasted into the target foods. Those concerned with transgenic modification of foods recognize that new toxins could be produced by the target foods, making them unhealthy or outright toxic to humans. Additional concerns include the potential for nutritional deficiencies, adverse nutritional changes and antibiotic resistance. A myriad of health problems are possible, according to some studies – many of them have occurred in test animals and humans, including negative effects on the testicles and reproduction in men and women, the immune system, blood cells, kidney, liver, pancreas and intestinal tract.

STUDY SUMMARY

"Genetically Modified Food — Great Unknown"

The study states that genetically modified foods create a threat to the health of the consumer. Transgenic plants contain DNA that is unstable, which makes it possible for foreign proteins and proteins that could contribute to allergies to synthesize. GMOs are digested much more slowly than their conventional counterparts, which could lead to alimentary canal diseases, as toxins in the foods, such as Bt toxin, are in the body for long periods of time. Roundup® pesticide is especially harmful when in the body, and can lead to cancer as it disturbs human hormonal metabolism.

2. WHO IS MONSANTO AND WHEN DID THEY START PRODUCING GENETICALLY MODIFIED FOODS?

Monsanto Company, an American multinational agricultural biotechnology corporation headquartered in Missouri, is a leading producer of genetically engineered seed. The company, founded in 1901 by John Francis Queeny, operated primarily as a major producer of plastics, including polystyrene and synthetic fibers. As a chemical company, notable achievements by Monsanto and its scientists include being the first company to mass-produce LEDs and performing breakthrough research on catalytic asymmetric hydrogenation. Products manufactured by the company deemed controversial include the insecticide DDT, PCBs (dielectric and coolant fluids) and Agent Orange. Monsanto is not known for its honesty or transparency regarding the dangers of DDT, PCBs and Agent Orange.

In 1983, Monsanto and three academic teams were the first to genetically modify a plant cell and conduct field trials of genetically modified crops. The first genetically modified food was the tomato. Between 1997 and 2002 the company came to focus heavily on biotechnology after a process of mergers and spin-offs. Monsanto pioneered the biotechnology industry by applying its business model to agriculture.

3. WHAT ARE THE CONCERNS ABOUT MONSANTO AND THEIR CLAIMS REGARDING GMO FOOD SAFETY?

The concern that I and a large percentage of the scientific, health care and environmental groups and the public have is that it may take decades to fully appreciate the negative impact of genetically modified food consumption upon the public. I have heard pro-GMO geneticists claim there is no evidence that GMOs pose a health threat because people have been eating GMOs since the 1990s, and if real dangers existed, people would be dropping like flies. I believe that this statement is a misrepresentation or at least it is not based upon careful scientific scrutiny: since the introduction of GMOs, people are experiencing an increased risk of various diseases including some cancers, gastrointestinal problems and autoimmune disease, just to name a few...people ARE dropping like flies. Who is to say that GMO consumption is not to blame, or is not at least a contributor to the deterioration of our health and environment? One cannot rule these possibilities either out or in at this point. In the meantime, I urge people to avoid GMOs until more scientific studies have examined their impact upon human health and our environment worldwide. To paraphrase Star Trek's Mr. Spock, when you eliminate the impossible, whatever remains, no matter how improbable, must be the truth.

Sex, Lies and Videotape

A major misrepresentation by Monsanto Company was that the safety and benefits of the ingredients in GMOs were well established. In fact, no long-term studies about either the safety or benefits of GMO ingredients exist. The FDA does not currently require safety studies of GMOs. This is a curious stance that I believe represents either ignorance or outright delusional thinking on the part of the decision-makers at the FDA. In fact, the FDA leaves the job of carrying out safety studies to Monsanto and other manufacturers of GMO products, resulting in inherently biased research and ultimately resulting in the largest uncontrolled study: the untested exposure of consumers to GM foods and non-food items such as cosmetics and medications. Some independent studies have already raised serious questions as to allergies, nutritional inadequacy and risks to our immune, renal, cardiovascular, hepatic and gastrointestinal systems. The conflict of interest here should be obvious, and a quote from George Orwell perfectly describes the problem: "The very concept of objective truth is fading out of the world. Lies will pass into history."

These and other potential health problems, which may not be obvious to physicians or the scientific community, could result from the consumption of GMO products. It should also be remembered that physicians uninterested in GMOs' potential health risks would not likely attribute various long-term health problems to GMO consumption. Said plainly, I doubt that the GMO-ignorant physician would recognize the possibility of a symptom or disease as having resulted from GMO consumption unless the patient was experiencing a health crisis unlike any other he or she had ever experienced, and this is unlikely.

Generally speaking, many mainstream physicians blindly trust the FDA, not questioning its contentions or the safety issues surrounding GMOs. Unless many people within a very short period of time develop acute symptoms from GMOs, as happened with the health supplement tryptophan, physicians probably would not recognize the connection of GMOs and their detrimental effects upon health. It is much more difficult to study, recognize and attribute the effects of foods on human health over the long haul. Nonetheless, with careful study it is possible to develop some conclusions about whether there are long-term health issues associated with GMOs. So far, limited but disconcerting evidence indicates there are! Please watch my interview on Fox (described in the Comment following Q. 33) that explores some of my media appearances on the Frankenfoods issue.

4. WHAT IS THE IMPACT OF GMO TECHNOLOGY ON OUR FOOD SUPPLY? WHAT ARE THE CONCERNS HELD BY OPPONENTS OF GMOS?

The impact of GMO technology on our food supply can be seen by the huge amount of commercialized GM foods that are sold around the country. First introduced to the food supply in the 1900s, GMOs are now present in the majority of processed foods in the U.S. GMOs are banned as food ingredients in Europe and other countries, but in the U.S., the FDA does not even require labeling of GMOs in food ingredient lists.

Currently, commercialized GM crops in the U.S. include sugar beets (95%), soy (94%), cotton (90%), corn (88%), zucchini and yellow squash (80%) and Hawaiian papaya (over 50%). Though there have been attempts to increase the nutritional benefits or productivity of food, the two main characteristics added to GMOs are tolerance to herbicides and ability of a plant to make its own pesticide. These changes have conferred no nutritional benefits on humans, only economic benefits for the seed manufacturers. Studies have shown an increased use of pesticide sprays, *not* less spraying as anticipated, or at least claimed, by the GMO industry. It is claimed that through GM technology, food can be modified to reproduce more quickly and with more desired traits. As for farmers producing higher crop yields, sadly this has not been demonstrated.

The public is increasingly concerned about human health and safety, partly in response to the dismissive attitude of the GM industry that perpetuates their "smarter than thou" attitude. The motivations of a pro-GMO "industrial complex" of biotech companies that produce GM seeds are clear. The public is no longer fooled by the strong lobbying attempts on the part of the GMO industry that insult our common sense and deny our freedom of choice to know and choose the health influences to which we are exposed. The disregard for the wants and needs of the public is apparent when the GM industry fights tooth-and-nail to prevent labeling of GMOs that would otherwise allow the public to choose what they want to eat. Why fight conducting appropriate safety studies? Why say the process of genetic modification of foods is identical to "natural selection" when it is not? Why claim we can solve the world's food shortage problem when the bigger problem is the delivery of food to those in need? These and other GMO myths I predict will perpetuate for years to come, driven by the seed manufacturers, politicians, lawyers and uninformed media. It is up to each individual to maintain a proactive attitude and a GMO-free lifestyle. The most powerful way to send a message that will change the GM industry is to refuse to eat their genetically manipulated foods.

5. HAVE GMOs BEEN PRODUCED, AS CLAIMED, WITH HIGHER NUTRITIONAL CONTENT COMPARED TO NON-GMOs?

Touted benefits of GMOs by proponents of GMOs include higher nutritional yields, less expensive food, food with medicinal benefits, and disease or insect resistant crops that require less herbicide or pesticide.

Nutritional Enhancement

There are strong doubts concerning the claim by GMO proponents that GMOs have either higher nutritional yield compared to non-GMOs or do not vary substantially in their level of nutrition. Genetic engineering has been used to increase the amounts of specific vitamins and nutrients in foods. This tactic, called nutritional enhancement, has been used to produce GM golden rice. This rice comes from a white rice crop inserted with the vitamin A gene from a daffodil plant. The vitamin level of the rice is beneficial in countries where there is a prevalent vitamin A deficiency.

A limited number of GMOs have enhanced nutritional content. Golden rice is currently the main nutritionally enhanced GM crop, although carrots have been created with more antioxidants, and bananas have been created with bacterial or rotavirus antigens. Researchers are currently focusing on prominent health problems like iron deficiency and the removal of proteins in foods that cause allergies.

One must be careful with haphazard nutritional manipulation of foods because not all of us will benefit from the added nutrition. The potential problems with GM nutrition enhancement include, but are not limited to:

- Nutritional toxicities can develop when one consumes foods with unnaturally enhanced nutritional content. Vitamin A toxicity results in a form of liver inflammation and enlargement called hepatitis. Even the water soluble nutrients such as vitamins B1 (thiamin), B2 (riboflavin), B3 (niacin), B5 (pantothenic acid) and B6 (pyridoxine) can result in toxicity when consumed in excess or imbalanced proportions.

- GMOs contain various anti-nutrients that can bind to certain nutritional factors (i.e., phytates) that render them non-absorbable. In other words, we are not what we eat, but what we absorb from what we eat. The concept of "nutritional equivalence," a term used by the GMO scientists to describe how GMOs' nutritional content matches up with their non-GMO counterparts, is false. GMOs are not nutritionally equivalent to non-GMO foods, as described elsewhere in this book.
- Consuming nutrients not based upon one's individualized needs can cause malabsorption of other nutrients because of competition among nutritional compounds. Malabsorption means that needed nutrition may not be fully absorbed in the body.

Personalized nutrition based on the unique needs of the individual can go a long way toward preventing and treating a wide variety of health problems. Unreliable nutritional supplementation, such as what may occur with GM nutrition enhancement, may cause more harm than good.

6. IS THERE ANY EVIDENCE THAT THE CONSUMPTION OF GMOS BY HUMANS IS UNHEALTHY?

There is much debate over the extent to which GMOs are healthy to consume. All GMOs currently sold in the U.S. have been approved by the government as healthy and safe for human consumption, but this does not mean that they are healthy or safe for human consumption. Remember, GMO "safety" studies and determinations are carried out by Monsanto and the seed manufacturers themselves – an inherently biased and self-serving strategy.

New Allergens, Increased Toxicity, Decreased Nutrition and Antibiotic Resistance

There are several types of potential negative health effects that could result from eating GMOs. The health effects of primary concern are: production of new allergens, increased toxicity, decreased nutrition and antibiotic resistance, just to name a few.

If the protein in a GMO comes from a source known to cause allergies, or from a source that is not generally consumed as human food, there is a concern that an allergic reaction could be elicited from the protein. Most plants produce substances that are toxic to humans. In a study on humans, one of the subjects in the experimental group showed an immune response to GM soy but not to non-GM soy. The GM soy contained a protein that was different from the non-GM soy. This finding showed that GMOs such as GM soy are capable of causing new allergies and can provoke immune reactions.

Fetuses Exposed to Toxic GMO Products

There is a legitimate concern that if a foreign or transgenic gene is inserted into a plant, toxins would be produced at higher levels, making the genetically modified plant dangerous for human consumption. This effect has been observed through conventional breeding methods of plants. A study conducted in Canada detected high levels of the protein Cry1Ab, found in GM Bt crops, circulating in the blood of pregnant women and their fetuses, and in the blood of non-pregnant women. It is unclear how the Bt toxin protein got into the blood; however, the study questions why GM Bt crops are being sold widely when research indicates serious concerns about the health and safety of GM products to both mother and fetus. The bottom line here is that pregnant women and their developing babies can suffer ill health effects from GMO products, including birth defects, impaired immune systems, and neurological and metabolic disorders. Unbelievably, the diet of a pregnant woman that includes GMOs may affect the genetic material of the developing fetus (gene expression), potentially affecting future generations by altering DNA (our genetic material) and through reproduction, passing on the damaged DNA.

Contaminated L-tryptophan

In 1989, 37 people died in the U.S. and 1,500 were permanently disabled from consuming L-tryptophan, an amino acid food supplement. As it turns out, the Japanese manufacturer of the tryptophan used a new manufacturing process involving GM bacteria without alerting any of its suppliers. The toxic tryptophan was produced at a single Japanese facility and sold in the U.S. under several different brand names – so at first it seemed that the tryptophan itself was the problem and not the GM bacterial contamination. The contaminated tryptophan caused some of those who consumed the amino acid to develop a serious condition called eosinophilia myalgia syndrome or EMS, an incurable condition that is often fatal, producing flu-like neurological symptoms. I was just a boy when my father, a chiropractor and nutritionist, had recommended tryptophan to a patient who then developed all of the symptoms of EMS and was seriously ill and hospitalized. At the time, my father could not have known that the problem was not the tryptophan, but the bacterially contaminated, GMO-tainted tryptophan.

The FDA claimed the tryptophan itself was the problem, when in actuality it was the bacterially-GMO processed tryptophan that caused the EMS. Tryptophan was removed from the commercial vitamin supplement market, even though tryptophan had been used without incident by hundreds of thousands of people without apparent incident. Eventually, tryptophan was allowed to return to the market, after years of public outcry forced the FDA to release its foothold on tryptophan. Many of those in the natural health care industry believed that the FDA had inappropriately blamed the supplement rather than the contamination process, using this example as justification to attack the vitamin industry as a whole.

The health effects of the GM bacteria-tainted tryptophan occurred fairly abruptly, allowing health authorities to quickly identify this health threat. In my experience, a public health epidemic must be obvious, severe and otherwise clearly demonstrate that a crisis is at hand before health authorities take action. Without an epidemic by this definition, public health issues often go unrecognized and/or are disguised as health problems that are diluted within a population's general health issues. The reason for the lack of clinical suspicion on the part of physicians is that they, generously speaking, are not thinking from a community-health mindset, but rather with a focus on individual patients, and are not considering GMO influences. With this mindset, I predict the medical community will fail to recognize and address both acute and chronic health problems stemming from GMO consumption, when proponents of GMOs claim that GMOs must be safe because they have been consumed by the public since the 1990s.

There are hundreds of examples of toxic compounds and microorganisms found in our food and water supply that may cause health problems ranging from cancer and infections to intestinal issues and even death. Some of these include E. coli bacteria, various parasites and drug-resistant gonorrhea. Toxic microorganisms and infectious agents inherent in our food supply pose health dangers that are compounded by the introduction of Frankenfoods. Allergens, toxins, altered gene expression and nutritional problems are just some of the health implications we chance by consuming GMOs.

Nutritional Content of GMOs

Frankenfoods are not "nutritionally equivalent" and assays have shown them to have poor nutritional value compared to their non-GMO counterparts. To make matters worse, our fruit, vegetable and grain crops have undergone unprecedented drops in nutritional content over the last few decades. A recent study comparing dozens of "wild-type" variety plants, those grown in the wild to the same species of plants grown on industrial farms, proved that the nutritional content of wild variety plants was dozens to thousands of times higher. It has also been known for years that organic plants have superior nutrition content compared with non-organic plant foods. Not surprisingly, significant nutritional losses have been shown in GM plants as well. GMO nutritional studies are scant at best, but assays that have been done show real diminished nutritional content — not superior nutritional content as claimed by pro-GMO advocates. The combinations of non-organic foods, industrially farmed foods and nutritionally compromised GMOs have paved the way for greater disease and disability.

Pro-GMO advocates say repeatedly that GMOs do not differ substantially from their non-GMO counterparts in nutritional quality. This claim has no basis as comprehensive nutritional tests have not been performed, and tests that have been carried out cast doubt upon the nutritional quality of GMOs. Individuals who are truly concerned with public safety would never release foods to the public that are considered or proven to be nutritionally inadequate compared to foods already on the market. GMOs have not been studied adequately for nutritional content. The limited study that has been done clearly shows GMOs are substantially different from non-GMOs. Some of the reasons for the nutritional inadequacy of Frankenfoods are outlined below.

Phytates

A gene inserted into a plant could cause that plant to produce a high level of phytate, a common compound found in seeds and grains that binds with minerals and makes them unavailable to humans, and decreases the nutritional and mineral value of the plant. Claims are made by GMO advocates that the nutritional value of GMOs is not substantially different from non-GMOs, but I believe this claim to be misleading. Even if the nutritional content of Frankenfoods was equivalent to non-GMOs, the higher phytate content would bind to the minerals, converting those minerals into forms that the body either cannot absorb as efficiently or cannot absorb at all. Also, the fact that GMOs contain higher phytate content means that they are not nutritionally equivalent. The current evidence suggests that GMOs are deficient in several nutrients, and it is suspected that GMOs also contain unnaturally high levels of phytates.

Phytoestrogens — Anticancer Compounds

A study done by Anita Bakshi in 2003 showed that a strain of genetically modified soybeans produced lower levels of phytoestrogen compounds. These compounds are believed to protect against heart disease, several autoimmune diseases and cancer. Phytoestrogens belong to a large group of natural phenolic compounds, with the three largest classes being the coumestans, prenylflavonoids and isoflavones. Phytoestrogens are not estrogen, but could act in the human body as weak estrogens or estrogen blockers, depending on what the body needs.

The accounts I have investigated regarding GMOs and lower concentrations of phytoestrogens are not precisely correct. GMOs seem to contain a reduced concentration of phytocompounds, not phytoestrogens. Phytocompounds are a large class of phyto- or plant compounds with many diverse, positive health benefits in the human body. Some of these phytocompounds can act as weak estrogens, progesterone and even testosterone. Others help tissues of the body heal from injury, or act as antioxidants, anti-cancer agents, immune regulators and detoxifiers. It is easy to predict that the reduced content of phytocompounds in our food supply will have a detrimental effect on the health of consumers, and at some point, maybe far into the future, manifesting as reduced quality and length of life.

Antibiotic Resistance

In recent years, health professionals and supervising agencies such as the Center for Disease Control (CDC) have begun to recognize the increasing number of bacterial strains that are resistant to antibiotics. Antibiotic resistance has become a major health crisis that might have been prevented had the medical community heeded the scientific evidence predicting we, as a society of "antibiotic over-consumers," would face an epidemic of antibiotic-resistant infections that would result in increased morbidity and mortality for current and future generations. Because of improper training and despite many warnings about the risk of antibiotics creating resistant strains even when used correctly, physicians have overprescribed antibiotics, leading to a worldwide pandemic antibiotic resistance. Antibiotic resistance has already resulted in both young and old people becoming resistant to many types of antibiotics by creating resistant genes. These resistant genes were produced when antibiotics, commonly and often inappropriately prescribed by doctors, were taken by the general population over the last few decades. People are now falling victim to infections, and perhaps even cancers and other diseases that might previously have been easily treated with appropriate antibiotics or other medications. There is concern that GMOs may potentially worsen this health crisis as GMO products may "jump" from GMOs in one's digestive tract and then "jump" or incorporate into the genes of the host — and we are the hosts!

Conceivably, bacteria living in the guts of humans and animals could pick up a gene resistant to antibiotics from a GM plant before the DNA is completely digested in the body. In fact, this phenomenon of gene-jumping from bacteria into humans was first described in 1959 and is known as Horizontal Gene Transfer (HGT). HGT is considered to be the primary reason for antibiotic or bacterial resistance. HGT is known to be responsible for antibiotic drug resistance passed on from one species to another bacterial species. Thus, eating a GMO containing antibiotic resistant bacteria could infect our DNA, in effect causing antibiotic drug resistance. GMO produced antibiotic resistance is not all that different from doctors overprescribing and incorrectly prescribing antibiotics to people, which caused the antibiotic dilemma in the first place. I predict that the pro-GMO industry will contribute to the present health crisis by promoting products that exacerbate the problem of antibiotic resistant bacteria. It is more critical than ever before to avoid GMOs, focus on healthy non-GMOs and practice healthy lifestyle habits — all toward maintaining optimal immune function. Given this problem, it's best to just say *NO* to Frankenfoods!

Many uneducated or misinformed people seem to believe GMOs are safe to eat because the government has approved them. What most people do not know is that the FDA does not assess the safety of GMOs and leaves safety studies and assessments up to the GMO industry itself. In the early days of the introduction of GM products to the market, the FDA "gave up" suspiciously easily on overseeing GMOs. Some of the reasons the FDA handed over our food safety to the GM seed manufacturers are reviewed throughout this book.

Most studies I have reviewed that claim GM crops are safe are industry linked and therefore biased. The few independent studies conducted on humans and the many studies conducted on animals involving the effects of consuming GM crops show many health risks. In a study where human volunteers were fed a single GM soybean, GM DNA survived digestive processing in the stomach and was detected in the digestive tract. Soybean DNA may prove to have the ability to be inserted into human DNA. Disrupted DNA is a necessary step towards aberrant health processes such as cancer, diabetes, autoimmune diseases and otherwise poor health.

Toxicity

A toxin is a substance that by definition is harmful to the human body. Toxins are ubiquitous, meaning toxins are found everywhere...inside and outside of the body. There is virtually no health condition or disease that does not involve some level of toxin accumulation and/or require detoxification. The process of detoxification occurs in most body cells and especially in the liver and gastrointestinal tract. The skin, lungs, cardiovascular system, kidneys and lymphatic organs also carry out detoxification.

Some toxins, known as exogenous toxins, by definition, enter the body from external environments, the foods we eat, the water we drink and the air we breathe. Yet other toxins are produced within the body, known as endogenous toxins. I do not believe that the current knowledge on the topic of GMOs is adequate to anticipate the toxin potential of GM crops. This topic deserves study before GMOs are made part of our daily diets. Concern regarding toxins is real, as theoretical toxin exposure from GMOs can arise from resistant bacteria that produce toxins themselves, pesticides produced by the GM food (e.g., corn) and disrupted DNA caused by the process of artificial gene insertion. Genetic manipulation of foods by definition produces unnatural and often unforeseen effects that could include increased toxin production and/or stronger plant toxins produced by GM crops themselves.

Incomplete and biased studies, DNA transfer, bacterial resistance, toxicity and reduced nutritional balance are just some of the concerns that demand further review and study. Until these and other concerns are addressed, GMOs should not be allowed into our food or non-food (i.e., medications and cosmetics) products.

7. HAVE THERE BEEN CLAIMS THAT GMO PRODUCTS HAVE CAUSED SPECIFIC HEALTH PROBLEMS IN HUMANS, INCLUDING AUTISM AND GASTROINTESTINAL DISORDERS? IS THERE ANY PROOF TO THESE ASSERTIONS?

Many researchers have been concerned about the links between GMO products and various health problems in humans. The prominence of autism, particularly in boys, was nowhere near as high 20 years ago as it is today. In 2008, 1 in 54 boys were found to suffer from ASD, or autism spectrum disorder, in the U.S. alone. In October 2011, Dr. Don Huber, a professor at Purdue University, gave a talk in which he described the physiological, behavioral and neurological symptoms identified in animals such as rats, pigs and cows that were fed GM feed. Autism specialists and physicians who attended the talk were shocked by the similarities between the symptoms of the animals eating GM feed and the symptoms of autistic children. Do similar symptoms imply a connection? No, but a connection has not been disproven either.

At this time, there is no known cause for autism. The predominant theory in Western medicine is that genetics is the biggest risk factor in the predisposition to autism. Virtually every gene-associated health issue is influenced by environment (i.e., diet) and other lifestyle factors, and autism is probably not any different. The timing of GMO introduction into the human food chain is too coincidental to dismiss as a potential influence upon the genetic expression of autism. Furthermore, I do not believe that the increase in autism and autism spectrum disorder diagnosis is solely responsible for the autism epidemic — the increased incidence of diagnosis — we are facing in the U.S. Some geneticists believe that not only is genetics a strong factor in determining susceptibility to autism, but also that environment and diet influence what is known as genetic expression — how, when and to what extent autism manifests in an individual. The timing of the introduction of GMOs into our food chain and the steady increase in special needs conditions begs an investigation. Foods are known to have both beneficial and detrimental effects, depending upon what is eaten and how the individual is affected by their chosen diet. People have been consuming GMOs for a relatively short time, but long enough to cause health problems. These health problems may be difficult to diagnose, particularly if doctors and GMO advocates will not even consider the potential for GMOs to cause adverse health effects.

In the studies Dr. Huber described, the animals were fed the same corn and soy on the market in the U.S. as for adults and children. Both GM soy and GM corn contain bacterial genes that have resistance to herbicides. Because of these bacteria, the GM corn and GM soy sold in the U.S. contain larger amounts of the toxic herbicide. Independent scientists who are finding the protein to not be as harmless to humans as Monsanto claims are researching the Bt toxin also found in GM corn. The rats used in the studies were found to be agitated and solitary. The same symptoms were found with the pigs. Veterinarian Don Skow described that his client's pigs, "would get cannibalistic...they would lose the ability to know where the feed was."

A significant number of autistic children also have gastrointestinal problems. A 2006 study reported that GI symptoms were elicited in 70% of children with ASD compared to 28% of children with typical development. Many GI disorders found in autistic children include imbalances in intestinal bacteria, inflammation and intestinal permeability. Health issues also resulted in a study in which animals were fed GMOs. The small intestines of GMO-fed livestock are much thinner than non-GMO fed animals. In a 1999 study published in the *Lancet*, rats fed GMO potatoes for 10 days were found to have severely altered cells in the lining of their stomachs and intestines. Since the introduction of GMOs into the U.S., the number of people contracting inflammatory bowel disease has increased by approximately 40%.

8. IS THERE A CANCER CONNECTION INVOLVING THE CONSUMPTION OF GMOS? WHAT ARE THE NEW COMPOUNDS (SPECIFICALLY RNA, DNA AND PROTEINS) NOT PRESENT IN NON-GMOS?

Numerous studies have shown a link between the consumption of GM products and the development of various types of cancer. A study performed in China in 2012 showed that plant microRNA, such as the GM parts containing Bt, was able to survive digestion and influence human cell function – so much for Monsanto's geneticists' claim that Bt does not pass beyond our stomach. This means that DNA can code for microRNA, which can be extremely dangerous and has been linked for years to human diseases including cancer and diabetes. A second study performed in 2013 showed that Bt or Cry-toxins found in GM crops contribute to blood abnormalities, including anemia, leukemia and other hematological malignancies (blood cancers).

Americans have the highest rate of cancer of any other nation in the world. One out of eight women in America has breast cancer, though only one out of ten are inherited. Nine out of ten incidences of breast cancer come from environmental triggers – including diet. It is simply unreasonable and unscientific to rule out the effect of GMO exposure on breast cancer and other diseases. I suspect that the reduction of healthful phytocompounds (phyto is the Greek word for plant) in Frankenfoods is one major factor of increased breast cancer incidence. The most significant factors that trigger breast cancer for women and men (yes, men can and do develop breast cancer) include the use of hormone replacement therapy (HRT), birth control pills, poor diet, stress, exposure to heavy metals (i.e., cadmium) and xenoestrogens (by-products of plastics manufacturing).

Both glyphosate and formaldehyde are found in GM products, specifically produce, but they are not found in non-GMOs. Novel RNA found in GMOs could be harmful to humans. Genetically modified foods introduce new combinations and mutations of DNA, which increase the chances of harmful RNA being produced accidentally and causing problems that could be passed on to future generations. Roundup® Ready soybeans, specifically, can produce unintentional variations of RNA. Bt is found in many GMOs, including soy products, corn and potatoes. Specific Bt toxins such as Cry1Ab can also be found in GMOs.

9. WHAT DOES MONSANTO CLAIM IS THE CAUSE OF THE INCREASED PREVALENCE OF SOME FORMS OF FOOD ALLERGIES SUCH AS SOY?

Monsanto claims there is currently no direct link between GMOs and allergies. Monsanto has stated that a likely reason for the increase in food allergies, specifically to soy, is due to greater consumption of soy in general, and not specifically GM soy. In the last two decades, there has been an upsurge in reporting of soy allergies in infants. Monsanto claims the infants' increased exposure to GM soy is not causing the increased allergy reports. They claim that the allergies are coming from more baby formula being made with soy and infants consuming too much during the growth and development years.

Monsanto has also pointed to the "hygiene hypothesis," which states that increased allergies come from infants and children being sheltered, causing an exaggerated response in those children when they are exposed to GMOs later in life. Before GMOs are released into the market, Monsanto tests both the physiochemical characteristics of proteins in the GMOs and the susceptibility of the introduced protein to digestion. However, all of the studies I have examined are designed improperly, focusing on artificial laboratory experiments meant to match a human being digestive response. These studies, in my opinion, fail to recreate the intricacies of not only the mammalian (human) digestive response, but the inherent and neurohormonal coordinated physiologic responses that go along with digestion. Simply put, a "fake stomach" in a laboratory can never recreate the normal digestive process, which makes this study's design and methodology flawed and essentially useless.

10. WHAT ARE THE PROTEINS THAT, WHEN INTRODUCED INTO CROPS, CAN INDUCE FOOD ALLERGIES?

Many studies have shown a link between the consumption of genetically modified foods and the development of mild to severe allergies. However, it is hard to identify a protein that could be a possible allergen before the product is actually consumed. A few proteins are often used to create GM products, and the GM crops themselves may have their protein and/or DNA structure altered, potentially creating GM foods with allergic potential. Also, GM foods sometimes are produced from genes from certain foods that, if an individual is allergic, would now increase one's risk of an allergic response. An example is the genetic modification of strawberries with Arctic fish. If an individual is allergic to fish, he/she may suffer an allergic reaction when eating strawberries. Many more examples of adverse GM combinations exist, posing health issues, and labeling laws do not keep up.

One of these proteins comes from Bt corn. The proteins that Bt creates, Bt Cry proteins, are used to stop an insect from feeding on crops by starving and killing the insect. It is claimed by GMO-pro geneticists as a whole that Bt Cry proteins are among the safest insecticides that can be used in agriculture. Their claim is that the protein is not expressed much, if at all, on the corn kernels themselves. Bt-corn industry promotes the concept that humans are not ingesting much of the protein at all when they ingest Bt corn. To claim that Bt Cry proteins are among the safest pesticides does not mean that they are safe or healthy for human consumption. This claim is analogous to the saying that dogs' mouths are among the cleanest of all mammals. This does not mean that dogs' mouths are clean – they're just cleaner than most dirty mammalian mouths! I believe that these Bt-proteins are harmful until proven otherwise, and any reputable scientist would do the public and its safety a service by disproving my assertion that Bt derived Cry proteins are unsafe.

The AFA3 protein has caused panic among consumers. This protein was found in the first GMO, the tomato plant, which was genetically engineered to resist frost. Scientists created this frost-resistant plant by injecting the antifreeze protein found in flounder into the plant seed. The antifreeze gene keeps flounder from freezing in cold waters. A person allergic to flounder could experience an allergic reaction after eating the antifreeze tomatoes. These tomatoes were never brought to the market.

It is possible that a genetically modified food could create an allergic reaction as a direct result of the genetic modification process. The person experiencing the allergic response could become confused if they had consumed a food that normally does not cause a reaction. The confusion is compounded because the adulterated proteins that provoked the allergic reaction are now found in GMOs, which differ from the non-GMO and normally non-allergic food counterpart. Research is continuing to examine the role of specific proteins found in GMOs and their link to allergies, inflammation and immune dysregulation, as well as other serious human health problems.

11. IS THERE ANY EVIDENCE THAT YOUNG GIRLS EXPOSED TO GM CROPS EXPERIENCE EARLY ONSET OF PUBERTY?

Studies have verified a link between hormones in genetically modified foods and early puberty in girls. Over the second half of the 20th century, the average age for girls to develop breasts dropped more than one year, and the average age for girls to get their first period decreased by months. Dr. Sam Epstein, chairman of the Cancer Prevention Coalition and author, believes there is a link between rBGH (found in genetically modified milk), early puberty and cancer. Consumers are concerned about the excess levels of hormones found in the milk.

Though Monsanto claims there is no link between the early onset of puberty in girls and increased consumption of GMOs, numerous studies have concluded there is indeed a link. The increased amount of hormones injected into GMOs is dangerous for young girls and increases their risk of early puberty, which can lead to cancer and other health problems.

12. IS THERE EVIDENCE TO SHOW THAT THE PESTICIDE PRODUCED BY GENETICALLY MODIFIED CORN CAN FIND ITS WAY INTO THE BLOOD OF PREGNANT WOMEN AND THEIR FETUSES?

Evidence has shown that toxins found in GM crops can also be found in the blood of all pregnant women and their fetuses. In a study published in *Reproductive Toxicology*, Aziz Aris and Samuel Leblac examined the blood of 30 pregnant women and 39 non-pregnant women to look for toxins found in GMOs, including glyphosate (Roundup), gluphosinate (herbicide), AMPA, 3-MMPA and Cry1Ab (Bt toxin). The study found no glyphosate or gluphosinate in the bloodstream of either group of women, but found 100% of 3-MMPA in the blood of the pregnant mothers and on the fetal cord, and 93% of Cry1Ab in the bloodstream of the pregnant mothers and 80% on the fetal cord.

STUDY SUMMARY:
"Hypothetical Link Between Endometriosis and Xenobiotics-Associated Genetically Modified Food"

Endometriosis, an inflammatory disease dependent on estrogen, affects approximately 10% of reproductive-aged women. This disease interferes highly with women's quality of life, as it often causes pelvic pain and infertility. An increasing amount of evidence points to environmental toxins as the cause of endometriosis. Xenobiotics may be found in GMOs posing long term safety risks, especially for women. The study further summarizes the toxic effects of xenobiotics, including glyphosate and Cry1Ab proteins, and explains the role of these toxins in the pathophysiology of endometriosis. A xenobiotic is a chemical found within an organism that is not normally produced by that organism and is not expected to be present and may cause varied health problems. Medications such as antibiotics are examples of xenobiotics found in our foods and water supply and prescribed by doctors.

13. IS THERE A POTENTIAL LINK BETWEEN THE BT PESTICIDE AND SUDDEN INFANT DEATH SYNDROME?

GMOs may cause numerous health problems in humans according to individual reports and studies. Many genetically engineered crops are modified to be herbicide and pesticide resistant, which causes the crops to contain higher levels of the poisonous herbicide or pesticide. The two main weed killers currently used by farmers are Roundup® and Liberty®. Both of these chemicals have antibacterial properties. Glyphosate, the active ingredient found in Roundup®, is known to also kill microorganisms in the intestine.

German research studies have shown that when Roundup® is part of a cow's diet, it causes the cow to have abnormal botulism growth. Botulism is a serious illness caused by bacteria that may live in improperly preserved or canned foods, or may enter the body through an exterior wound. An apparent cause of botulism poisoning in livestock is the overuse of Roundup®, especially on Roundup® Ready Crops. The ingestion of Roundup® could have the same effect on humans. Low levels of botulism are also associated with sudden infant death syndrome, or SIDS. The increased overuse of Roundup® could have very serious implications for infants if pregnant women are ingesting the toxic chemicals that normally control botulism growth and prevent botulism poisoning but also kill the beneficial bacteria.

14. WHAT IS THE PROCESS OF GENETIC MODIFICATION OF FOODS (TRANSGENIC MODIFICATIONS)?

There are eight main steps involved in developing GM crops:

1. **First, the gene of interest is isolated.** It is necessary to have existing knowledge of the structure, location, and/or function of a gene on a chromosome to identify the specific gene responsible for a desired trait in an organism. For example, desired traits for GMO plants include tolerance to drought or resistance to insects.

2. **After isolating the gene, it is inserted into a transfer vector.** Most commonly, a plasmid, or circular model of DNA, is used to transfer the isolated gene from the naturally occurring soil bacterium. Using rDNA, the gene of interest is inserted into the plasmid.

3. **The modified cell containing the plasmid and the new gene are combined with cells from the original plant**, and some of the cells take up the plasmid containing the transfer DNA.

4. **After transformation, genes responsible for resistance are inserted into the plasmid** and are transferred along with the genes containing the desired traits.

5. **When the cells are exposed to an antibiotic, herbicide, etc.,** only the transformed cells survived.

6. **The transformed cells can then be regenerated** to form entire plants by culturing tissue.

7. **After GMO plants are grown, tests are performed** to determine the number of copies of the gene inserted, whether or not the copies are intact, and whether or not the gene is functional.

8. **Assessments of the food and environmental safety of the GMOs are also conducted** (albeit biased, superficial, misrepresented and inadequate) in connection with testing of plant performance.

Many claims have been made and concerns have been raised about studies that have shown nutritional differences between non-GMO plants and GMO plants produced as a result of unnatural genetic manipulation. Long-term epidemiological studies have not been performed to determine safety in humans or animals. According to some anti-GMO, pro-health groups, authors and scientists, toxic products, nutritional irregularities, bacterial resistance and the effects of changing the gene sequence of the target food have not at all been firmly established as safe for humans and the environment. An entire population has been exposed to untested GMOs, resulting in ill health effects in human study subjects and observations by farmers of serious health impacts on various body systems of test animals. It is reasonable to suspect, given the early reports and studies to date, that Frankenfoods are dangerous.

15. HOW DOES TRANSGENIC MODIFICATION OF FOODS DIFFER FROM NATURAL SELECTION AGRICULTURAL METHODS OF FOOD PRODUCTION?

In many industrialized countries, including the United States, there is little genetic diversity within a given crop of food. However, farmers in more agricultural societies such as China, Ethiopia and the Near East have been using traditional farming methods for many years, mutating their crop outcomes by replanting seeds. Farmers have taken seeds from crops that can be used for various benefits, such as using the corn seed for tortilla flour, roasting corn or popcorn. These farmers have also learned that by replanting seeds from specific seasons, they can expect a different crop outcome. Crops in less industrialized countries, though they have been modified naturally by farmers replanting seeds, still have greater genetic biodiversity than those currently found in industrialized nations such as the U.S.

Monsanto has claimed the transgenic gene manipulation used to produce GMOs is identical to natural biodiversity and natural selection, as I have described it above. I am convinced that this claim is false and misleading. In nature, one would never see the result of a tomato "having sex" with a fish, but this is an example of transgenic research. Corn would never produce toxic pesticides in nature nor would salmon genes find their way into strawberries. Genetic manipulation uses a gene gun that blasts the desired gene into the host seed, causing unnatural alterations in the food that may affect the health and natural course of biodiversity that would otherwise occur naturally. No reputable geneticist or biologist would ever claim that the gene gun method of transgenic gene manipulation is identical to natural selection — nature's method of modifying foods during the course of plant evolution. Such a claim of equivalency between transgenic and natural methods is a lie meant to mislead and confuse an uneducated public about the difference between these methods and the potential health risks and environmental impacts.

Natural selection also plays a role in the modification of foods and the outcome of a crop. In any generation or any crop cycle, more seeds are produced as offspring. As in any offspring, generations of a seed have variations. Some variations of the seeds are due to heredity, and some result from natural mutation. Seeds with more favorable traits survive more prosperously and reproduce to create a generation with a stronger gene pool of favorable traits. It seems reasonable, as claimed by geneticists, that transgenic gene modification could result in more resistant crops against changing weather conditions. However, nature has already proven the ability to naturally bio-diversify crops, but transgenic manipulation has not. There is a concern that if a GMO crop that has been manipulated to withstand certain environmental conditions, like extreme cold, is exposed to extreme heat, then that crop might fail as a direct result of genetic manipulation. In effect, the GMO process has created a food product that is not flexible enough to withstand unpredictable environmental conditions. GMO crops designed to genetically withstand certain environmental conditions, such as insects, weather or chemicals, may be far weaker at withstanding certain types of environmental, insect and toxin exposures.

Transgenic modification of foods is very different from the traditional methods of farming and genetic modification of a crop, and from natural selection with no human intervention. When natural selection plays a role in the outcome of a generation of a crop of wheat, for example, genetic diversity is abundant, although seeds with a specific genetic composition are more likely to survive than others. GMO wheat, however, is modified so that an entire generation of seeds has the same set of DNA. Because of this, some seeds do not have the ability to survive over others when environmental changes occur, like seeds would with a more diverse gene pool. Thus, an environmental change will cause the seeds of a crop of GMO wheat to either fully survive or be wiped out entirely.

16. WHAT ARE THE MOST COMMON GENETICALLY MODIFIED FOODS?

The Flavr Savr Tomato

The tomato was the first widespread genetically modified food in the U.S. GMO tomatoes, particularly the Flavr Savr tomato, were a very popular product for about four years until the scientist who created the GMO tomato expressed on television his concerns about whether the GMO tomatoes could be carcinogenic. This led to bans of GMOs at major food chains and of the Flavr Savr tomato. It seems that Monsanto, the FDA and various agencies involved in allowing GMOs to make their way into the food chain have not changed and continue to put the public at risk. Even if GMOs are eventually proven safe, that should not negate the need to have a GMO approval process in place. As it stands now, the FDA has placed the entire burden of proof of safety of GMOs in the hands of Monsanto and other GMO seed manufacturers themselves. This level of blind trust by the FDA that allows genetically modified seed manufacturers to police themselves has predictably resulted in many questionable practices in the areas of human health, environmental safety and political action.

The Hawaiian Papaya

The papaya is an example of a GMO that seems to have had a beneficial environmental impact. The papaya is a popular GMO food in Hawaii due to the ringspot virus, which was a serious problem in the Hawaiian papaya industry. In the 1980s, papayas were genetically modified to be resistant to the virus that would likely have obliterated the entirety of Hawaii's papaya crop. The example of the Hawaiian papaya is perhaps the only example of a clear environmental benefit, at least in the short term, of GMO manipulation of a food to prevent an agricultural catastrophe. This acknowledgement does not change the potential for the GMO papaya, and other GMOs, to have harmful effects upon both the environment and human consumption. Currently, the United States and Canada allow for transgenic papayas to be sold at large.

Rice, Potatoes and Bt-Corn

Rice is one of the top genetically modified foods being researched throughout the world, with the goal of making it resistant to pests. Potatoes are also being genetically modified and sold with the intention of being grown and sold as starch potatoes. Approximately 10% of potatoes found in supermarkets today are genetically modified.

Corn is also a major genetically modified product in the U.S. However, because corn is wind-pollinated, GMO corn may be affecting unmodified strains due to winds spreading GMO seed and contaminating corn in other countries such as Mexico and possibly the United States. A variety of corn known as Bt-corn has been genetically modified to produce its own pesticide toxin, intended to kill the insects that feed upon the corn. It is claimed that the Bt-corn breaks down in the stomach of humans and thus cannot cause harm. Rigorous studies examining the safety of human consumption of Bt-corn have not been carried out. However, some studies indicate many serious health problems in humans who were fed Bt-corn, suggesting the Bt-corn either does not break down, or incompletely breaks down, in the stomach of human beings. Also, beyond the stomach, toxins such as pesticides (i.e., Bt-toxins) require both intestinal and liver detoxification. No mention of the detoxification process was mentioned in any of the studies of Bt-toxin metabolism in humans.

Bt-Corn, Digestion and Detoxification

As a clinician who routinely deals with patients with intestinal issues, I can tell you with 100% certainty that people with and without known gastrointestinal issues vary greatly in their ability to digest and detoxify toxins in the environment. I have found that a large percentage of my patient population fails to produce adequate stomach acid and pepsin, two essential digestive juices produced by the stomach. These digestive juices are partly responsible for transforming various environmental toxins, such as pesticides, so they can be fully detoxified by the liver. To claim that human beings are inherently capable of digesting Bt-toxin found in corn is a dangerous claim, as it assumes that all people digest and detoxify normally – in fact, we do not! Depending upon the type of pesticide or toxin in question, the intestinal tract, liver and kidneys may play a role in the accumulation and detoxification of the toxin into forms that can be readily eliminated from the body.

As of the time of this writing, I have found no evidence that baseline determinations of digestive and detoxification capacity have been carried out. With no baseline metabolic functions, any claims of safety of Bt-toxin are simply unsubstantiated. My experience with hundreds of patients over the last 25 years suggests a high prevalence of inadequate digestive and detoxification abilities and a strong susceptibility of the average person to accumulate many environmental toxins. I further suspect that Bt-toxin poses health threats to humans and other mammals, impacting virtually every cell and major organ system of the body.

Bt-Corn and the Stomach

What if the Bt-pesticide does not break down in the stomach? Many people have low levels or no stomach acid or digestive enzymes, creating the possibility that the Bt-toxin would not be broken down before it reaches the circulation. It seems neither the seed manufacturers nor the FDA have conducted studies of real people who may not digest perfectly or who have health conditions that might affect how they digest or metabolize toxins such as Bt-pesticide. In one study, people fed Bt-corn showed changes in their gastrointestinal tracts characteristically seen in the guts of those with malabsorption syndromes, many autoimmune diseases and gastrointestinal disorders. Farmers have also observed in animals the same changes in the gastrointestinal tract and other organs that the human study showed.

Genetically Modified Soy

Of all crops, soy is the most heavily modified. More than half of the world's soy was genetically modified in 2007. In general, anyone eating soy or soy products in the U.S. is eating at least partially genetically modified material. GM soy contains far fewer phytochemicals that can help treat and prevent many health problems, including hormonal related cancers. Soy products, once very popular among health conscious consumers, are being avoided because of concerns about health safety. The effects of soy on the thyroid gland, growth and development of children, and cancer might actually be a result of the GMO soy and not from naturally farmed soy. The point is that no one knows, and until we do know, our food supply should remain Frankenfood-free!

"Got Contaminated Milk?"
Recombinant Bovine Growth Hormone

Milk is currently one of the most controversial GMOs due to the addition of recombinant bovine growth hormone (rGBH) into milk. This hormone allows for higher milk yields to be produced, as the mammary cells that enable cows to produce milk are kept alive longer than normal. When used incorrectly, as it is now in the cattle industry, rGBH can cause an increased rate of cancers and other health problems in cows, humans and other mammals. Growth hormone or its derivative IGF1 (insulin-like growth factor), also known as somatomedin-C, has been found in cow's milk in various studies.

One study of milk production of cows given rBGH claimed the amount of the hormone found in cow's milk was "inconsequential" to human health. One problem with this statement is that they measured the wrong indicator: they measured growth hormone and not IGF1. In fact, all reputable medical studies measure IGF1, as this measurement is known to be reliable. Growth hormone is not accurately measured in cow's milk because it breaks down too quickly. IGF1 is a much more stable form of growth hormone and can be accurately measured. The authors of this study incorrectly concluded that the amount of growth hormone found in the milk of cows fed rBGH was too low to cause health concerns. There is simply no basis for this statement, because any amount, in a susceptible person, can cause serious health problems. The fact that any growth hormone in any form was found in cow's milk poses a potential health threat to humans in the short- and long-term. Those who drink milk and consume dairy products are at risk of detrimental health effects affecting many cells, tissues and organ systems. Some health problems that may result from ongoing exposure to rBGH in cow's milk include cancers like leukemia; hyperinsulinemia; muscle, joint and nerve pain; carpal tunnel syndrome and high cholesterol. Growth hormone found in our foods in varying amounts and forms does not carry the potential health benefits that properly monitored growth hormone provided by physicians can yield.

Canola Oil and Aspartame

Canola oil and Aspartame are among the most abundant of all GMOs. In Canada, approximately 80% of canola crops are genetically modified. The rapeseed, the source of canola oil, is modified to be more resistant to herbicides. Modified rapeseed also produces one of the main pollens used to make honey. Some Aspartame, an artificial sweetener, contains bacteria modified to boost its yield. Canola oil, Aspartame and rapeseed are found in hundreds of foods as ingredients and are extremely difficult, but not impossible, to avoid if one wishes to reduce the intake of GMOs.

Known GMOs

GMOs are now pervasive within the American food supply. Even with diligent efforts, avoiding GMOs is difficult and may eventually become an impossible task if the GMO seed manufacturers and various government and industry supports continue with their GMO agendas. Sadly, those of us who wish to avoid GMOs must maintain a high degree of diligence reading labels, trusting those labels and purchasing foods presumably GMO free. Evidence also suggests that foods known to be non-GMO may be cross-contaminated with GMOs. Compounding the difficulties of maintaining a GMO-free lifestyle, labeling regulations are at best incomplete, forcing consumers to just "do their best" and hope their quality of health and length of life are not adversely affected. Following is a list of some of the more common GM foods and products:

- Rapeseed
- Papaya
- Honey
- Squash
- Rice
- Red-hearted chicory

- Soybean
- Cottonseed oil
- Sugar cane
- Tobacco
- Tomatoes
- Meat

- Corn
- Peas
- Sweet corn
- Vegetable oil
- Canola

- Sugar beets
- Potatoes
- Dairy products
- Flax
- Vitamins

For a more detailed list, see Question 23.

Many websites and a few books exist that expand upon this list and offer recipes to make preparing GMO-free foods easier, including my book due out in 2014, *The GMO-free Gluten-free Weight Loss Solution.* Familiarize yourself with the growing list of GMO crops, foods and food products so that you can avoid such items. Food preparation and eating at restaurants will become increasingly difficult, but not impossible. My upcoming book provides dozens of GMO-free and gluten-free recipes. Later in this book I have provided ten days of gluten-free and GMO-free daily food choices and some recipes to get you started. Please consult my upcoming book for many more recipes and food choices as part of my longevity plan. Follow me on Twitter @DrMichaelWald and Facebook for more GMO-free and gluten-free recipes and food plans.

17. WHAT ARE GMO PROTEINS? WHAT ARE THE HIGHLY PROCESSED DERIVATIVES OF GMO THAT CONTAIN LITTLE OR NO DNA PROTEIN, THOUGHT BY SOME TO POSE HEALTH RISKS?

GMOs may contain GMO proteins. I use the term "GMO proteins" to refer to the unnaturally created proteins resulting from genetic manipulation of seeds by biotech companies like Monsanto. Proteins, especially those that are unnatural or "foreign," like some of the proteins that are contained in GMOs, may provoke immune responses. The immune system is designed by nature to recognize foreign substances, including proteins. Pro-health groups and anti-GMO advocates are concerned that the consumption of GMO proteins may eventually be proven to pose health risks.

Proteins are made of individual amino acids. The types of amino acids and their order or sequence determine what food it is. The order of amino acids in a steak, for example, is different from soy protein, which differs from fish protein. These different protein sources are determined by their special protein sequences. GMOs have artificially engineered protein sequences. Geneticists will claim that GMO proteins are identical to those of the non-GMO crop proteins. This is clearly a lie, because a laboratory technology known as polymerase chain reaction (PCR) is used by farmers to identify GMO crops from non-GMO crops. It is my contention that the proteins found in GMOs can potentiate autoimmune disease, promote inflammation and potentially cause other adverse health effects.

GMO proteins are not the only aspect of GMOs that create concern among anti-GMO advocates, including myself. The absence of GMO protein does not mean there is no potential for harm from their consumption, as is claimed by pro-GMO geneticists. The highly processed derivatives of GMO containing little or no DNA protein are lecithin, vegetable oil, cornstarch and starch sugars, including syrups, and sugar. Corn oil and soy oil, which are free of DNA and protein, are sources of lecithin, which is widely used in processed foods as an emulsifier. There is very little, if any, DNA (genetic material) or protein from the original GMO crop in vegetable oil. Vegetable oil is made of triglycerides, and the refining process removes nearly all non-triglyceride ingredients. But the absence of protein or DNA from such oil, which according to some studies includes some GM food products, should not imply that health risks do not arise from other aspects of the GMO manufacturing process. Gene transfer, antibiotic resistance, toxins and nutritional problems are also potential sources of concern, beyond the potential health risks of GMO-produced proteins that I have addressed throughout this book.

The DNA of GMOs

The changes to a GMO's DNA may cause the production of new or known toxins, cause nutritional issues or affect the gene expression of the food's genes, provoking any number of health issues. Gene up-regulation, the increased expression of genes, or down-regulation, the decreased expression of genes, cannot be accurately predicted, and up-regulation of cancer genes (oncogenes) cannot be ruled out as a danger of GMOs: these genes may somehow transfer from the foods into our own bodies. Some scientists have confirmed that DNA can "jump" from the food to our intestinal bacteria and can potentially affect our health adversely by the phenomenon known as Horizontal Gene Transfer (HGT). Furthermore, intestinal bacteria may make their way into the general circulation through the small intestine lining — a phenomenon known as "bacterial translocation" (BT) — precipitating health problems throughout the body. GMO geneticists have denied that HGT can occur with GMOs, but HGT was proven to occur with GMOs decades ago. Today, consumers are buying and eating GMOs daily without knowing the potential health risks.

Pusztai's Rat Study

Former Scotland Rowett Research Institute's Arpad Pusztai researched extensively the health risks of GMOs. Pusztai's research concluded that rats fed genetically modified potatoes were seen to have smaller livers, hearts, testicles and brains. He also concluded that the rats had damaged immune systems and structural changes in their white blood cells, which made them more vulnerable to disease and infections as compared to rats being fed non-GMO potatoes. Thymus and spleen damage was also seen, as well as enlarged tissues, including tissue in the pancreas and intestines, and cases of liver atrophy and significant proliferation of stomach and intestine cells. All of these problems were also signs of greater future risks of cancer. These results showed up merely 10 days after testing was done, and persisted after 110 days, the human equivalent of 10 years.

It may not be possible to adequately perform human studies because the possible health issues associated with GMOs may look like the health issues we, as a population, are currently experiencing. The rise in special needs health issues including autism, hyperactivity, certain cancers, autoimmune and infectious diseases are associated with the introduction of GMOs over the past 10-20 years. Although a causal relationship has not been proven, or even attempted to be proven, an association between the introduction of GMOs and these and other health problems cannot yet be ruled out.

Genetic Roulette

Jeffery M. Smith's 2007 book, *Genetic Roulette: The Documented Health Risks of Genetically Engineered Foods* describes in some detail Pusztai's study. When a transgenic gene functions in a new cell, it may produce different proteins than are intended. These proteins produce chemicals that include cellular messengers, molecules that signal other cells to alter their function. There is a real concern that abnormal cellular expression could result from these molecules produced by transgenic processes, causing cancer, autoimmune diseases and other health problems. There is simply no way to know the potential harmful effects of these proteins without scientific research, and no research has been conducted yet to assess this issue.

There is also concern over health risks of Bt toxin produced by corn. Some farmers use a pesticide protein called Bt toxin as a spray for GM corn crops. People exposed to the spray have been seen to develop allergy-like symptoms, and mice having ingested the protein have developed strong immune responses and excessive cell growth, a process that occurs in cancers. A growing number of human and livestock illnesses have also been linked to Bt crops.

18. ARE THERE ANIMAL PRODUCTS THAT HAVE BEEN GENETICALLY MODIFIED AVAILABLE FOR HUMAN CONSUMPTION?

Modified plants are rapidly becoming popular throughout the world, but the same cannot be said for genetically engineered animals. Though there has been a great amount of testing of genetically modified plants, the genetic engineering of animals has been a slow and extremely expensive process. However, researchers have been exploring the possible benefits of GM animals. The modification of animals is being perfected, which is predicted to transform GM research.

Although genetically modified animal meat is restricted from much of the commercial market, GM bacteria and other GMOs have been fed to animals to affect their milk and even their excrement. For example, GM pigs have been modified to excrete waste that is more environmentally friendly. The U.S. Food and Drug Administration, which regulates GM animals, has yet to approve GM livestock for agricultural use. However, it is predicted that GM animals will be as widespread as non-GM animals in approximately 20 years, starting in China and Cuba, and then coming to the United States and Europe.

Omega-3 Fatty Acids in Pork

The potential benefits of pigs excreting friendlier environmental waste and their meat containing higher omega-3 fatty acid content is certainly appealing, but unforeseen health effects must also be studied. As a clinical nutritionist, I also find it interesting that the GM industry is exploring, at great expense, incorporating omega-3 fatty acids into pig meat. For years the FDA and mainstream medicine have been overwhelmingly against adding nutritional supplements like omega-3 fats to a "well-balanced diet" in spite of the abundant scientific evidence suggesting their short- and long-term health benefits. Omega-3 fats are healthy fats with decades of positive research. The same extensive research has not been carried out on GMOs fed to animals. As a nutritionist, I am well aware of the significant health benefits of omega 3 fatty acids. What I am not at all confident about is if the omega-3s processed genetically are "nutritionally equivalent" to non-GMO omega-3s.

The AMA and FDA Anti-Nutritional Supplement Stance

Farmers and seed technologists know full well the benefits of omega-3 fatty acids on the yields of livestock. It will be very telling to see whether the FDA approves GM animal production because, if they do, the approval would have to ignore both the FDA's and the AMA's (American Medical Association) anti-nutritional supplement stand. There is a difference between consuming pork modified with omega-3 fatty acids and taking omega-3 nutritional supplements. Supplements can be provided by a health care provider based on a person's health goals and blood tests. When one eats the omega-3s artificially placed within pig meat, the amount of omega-3 will vary from pig to pig and cannot be tailored to the unique omega-3 needs of the individual. An actual danger of omega-3 fats added to pig meat is that people who are taking blood thinners such as aspirin or Coumadin might experience excessive bleeding when their omega-3 intake is increased. Also, pork must be cooked thoroughly to avoid parasites and other infectious diseases. Heating omega-3s during the cooking process converts potentially healthful omega-3 unsaturated fatty acids into dangerous saturated fatty acids. Nutritional supplementation of meat should rarely be attempted as a standard practice if one wishes to avoid incorrect nutritional supplementation.

19. IS THERE A WAY TO DETECT GMOS SCIENTIFICALLY, SUCH AS TESTING FOR DNA CONTENT?

Currently, there are two methods to test for the presence of GMO in plants, seeds and other food ingredients: the ELISA protein antibody test and the protein strip test. These tests, used mainly to help farmers separate their GM grain from their non-GM grain, require only a small investment for equipment and personnel and allow for relatively quick turnaround times. However, a disadvantage of the ELISA and protein strip tests are that they detect only specific proteins, such as Bt or RR, which are not always readily available. Thus, these tests are not useful to detect certain GMO proteins in a food or plant. The phenomenon of *not* detecting GMO proteins with a food or plant when proteins *are* present is known as a false-negative. False-negative test results will allow GMO proteins to make their way into the plants and then to the bellies of the general public. False-positive protein tests are also likely to occur based on the limitations of the testing technologies employed.

DNA tests using polymerase chain reaction (PCR) technology are also helpful in making decisions regarding the separation of grain crops, and are often used for decisions involving breeding, marketing and production. The PCR method is generally recognized as the most accurate method. With all of these tests, false-positives and false-negatives are rare, but they do occur. A major advantage of PCR detection is that accurate PCR testing helps quantify the percentage of GMO from non-GMO samples.

In summary, PCR technology is considered the most accurate method of detecting GMO contamination, which is essential for the consumer to make informed food health and safety choices.

STUDY SUMMARY:

"Detection and Traceability of Genetically Modified Organisms in the Food Production Chain"

This study discusses the current issue of labeling and traceability of genetically modified products on the market. Currently, the EU requires labeling of foods containing detectable transgenic material. However, proposed legislation would extend labeling to foods containing no trace of genetically modified material. The new legislation would also impose a new system of labeling and traceability of the food and feed manufacturing system. Implementing such legislation would force producers of GM food and feed to sample their products and repeatedly assess them for any changes in structure.

Currently, analyzing GMOs focuses on either the transgenic DNA inserted or the novel protein(s) expressed. For most DNA-based detection methods, a polymerase chain reaction is used. For most protein-based methods of analysis, enzyme linked immunosorbent assays with antibodies binding the novel protein are used. New methods of detection are also being introduced, including the use of microarrays, mass spectrometry and surface plasmon resonance. However, there are many challenges in GMO detection, including the detection of transgenic material in organisms with varying chromosome numbers.

Traceability systems document a product's history, identifying potential food safety problems before the products reach the market, protecting us from being sold contaminated food. In these systems, there are particular requirements for each step in the chain of food processing. The feasibility of these systems depends on many factors, including permissible levels of contamination and detection methods. Much progress has been made in the fields of traceability, sampling and detection. However, some issues remain unresolved, and future success with these systems will rely heavily on legislation.

Author's note: I believe it would have been prudent to develop far more reliable and reproducible GMO detection methods before GMOs were placed in our pantries. Now, sadly, it is too late – GMOs can never be removed from our environments entirely due to cross-contamination. The best we can do at this point is to stop this problem from continuing to mount.

20. WHAT IS PCR TESTING AND HOW HAS IT BEEN APPLIED TO FOODS FOR THE IDENTIFICATION OF GMO CROPS?

Polymerase Chain Reaction (PCR) is a laboratory technique where pieces of DNA can be copied, or amplified, so they are more easily and accurately detected in a testing sample. PCR testing has been in widespread use in medicine for years and is very useful, but like all laboratory technologies, can yield false positives and false negatives.

PCR is a technique to amplify a piece of DNA by using in vitro enzymatic replication. Scientists in GMO research use PCR to detect specific segments of DNA with genes for traits that the researchers are trying to make more prominent in their GMOs, such as a gene for a natural herbicide or pesticide, or a gene resistant to a certain disease. In the PCR process, a specific sequence of DNA containing the desired gene is detected and cut out of its longer sequence. That DNA sequence then serves as a template for replication. A chain reaction takes place where the DNA template is amplified exponentially. Using PCR, a single or a few copies of DNA can replicate to generate millions or more copies of the original DNA sequence.

PCR is easily relatable to the identification of GM crops. An organism genetically modified to have a specific trait, such as a high resistance to disease, can often be identified as a GM product using PCR testing. PCR testing involves using an agarose gel run alongside a DNA size marker with DNA bands for which the sizes are known. The template DNA run in the gel will be longer in length than the PCR DNA. The template DNA will also run more slowly through the gel and appear as a band closer to the top of the gel. Primers, which are put on the ends of segments of DNA used in PCR, will be shorter, run faster and create smears of DNA closer to the bottom of the agarose gel.

PCR technology is clearly very complex, but the test strips are easy to use to detect GMO products in various feed samples.

21. WHAT ARE THE CURRENT GOVERNMENT REGULATIONS REGARDING GMO AND FOOD LABELING?

The regulation of genetically modified foods has been one of the most recent trade battles between the United States and Europe. According to the U.S. government, there are specific reasons for which organisms are allowed to be genetically modified:

- To delay ripening of food
- To delaying rotting of food
- To prolong the shelf life of certain foods in stores
- To add color to natural fibers before harvesting
- To reduce the need for fertilizers
- To increase resistance to pests and fungi
- To increase the effectiveness of herbicides on harmful weeds

Two main distinctions exist between Europe and the United States regarding GMOs: (1) the approval of GMOs by safety regulatory monitors; and (2) the labeling of GMO products. The FDA is responsible in the U.S. for approving GMOs under the Food, Drug, and Cosmetic Act of 1992 (FDCA). The FDCA authorizes the FDA to remove any food from the food supply that contains any poisonous substances that might render the food hazardous to health if consumed. GMO products containing additives not generally recognized as safe are required to have a safety review.

In Europe, a company must request approval from their food safety authority if they intend to manufacture or import a GM product. In the U.S., the FDCA requires in Section 403 that "consumers must be informed, by appropriate labeling, if a name no longer applies to the new food, or if a safety or usage exists to which consumers must be alerted." However, the FDA does not believe it is necessary to label a food product with the presence of genetically modified material. The majority of other countries endorsing GM products in the commercial market follow labeling policies similar to those of the U.S., such as:

- The FDA does not require labeling of GMOs as a mandatory practice. This is an entirely voluntary process and loosely regulated.

- If a food says "100% Organic," then it is supposed to be GMO-free up to 0.01% of GM ingredients (meaning it may still contain some GM products). If the food says "Organic," then it may be as high as 90% GMO-free. If the food says "Made with Organic Ingredients," then it may be up to 70% GMO-free.
- If a food says it does not contain certain ingredients, such as soy, corn or canola, then it should be free of these GMOs.

I can speak from personal experience producing various nutritional products that labeling requirements are far too loose to be trusted. I used to produce a health bar where the supplier of raw ingredients would have placed "GMO-free" or virtually anything else that I wanted on the product label. I was given conflicting information regarding what I could claim on the label by a bar manufacturer, and they said very plainly to me that I could put anything I wanted on my label. In fact, this same company contacted me one day and told me that they ran out of my organic rice ingredient, but they would gladly replace it with organic pea protein. I explained that the problem with this was that not only would the taste of the bar change, but we would have to change the labels, website and other marketing materials. They responded with a statement similar to, "No, we can just put the pea protein in." Once I realized the uselessness of the current labeling laws and integrity of some food manufacturers, I discontinued the entire production of my health bar. I was not at all comfortable with placing statements on the health bar that were inaccurate and untrue.

What You Don't Know, You Don't Know

Labeling is an absolute necessity for public safety. People need to know what they are consuming. If we become lax about labeling, then we cannot make educated philosophical and health decisions regarding our food choices. How will the vegan or vegetarian know if their food fits their choices? How can the person with a fish allergy ever eat pork or strawberries that may have been genetically modified to contain fats and proteins from fish? The public must have the ability to make personal and smart food choices.

The GM, or what I prefer to call the Frankenfood, industry is working hard to take this freedom away from the public. In 2013, after U.S. chemical giant Monsanto and other food manufacturers spent millions of dollars to defeat a California proposition that would have made GMO labeling mandatory, protestors began a "March Against Monsanto" movement to demonstrate against GMOs and Monsanto. The *Washington Post* reported in January 2014 that two states, Maine and Connecticut, have passed legislation requiring GMO labeling; laws will go into effect after nearby states pass similar legislation. The National Conference of State Legislatures reports that similar legislation has been introduced in 30 states in 2014. However, Monsanto has threatened to sue states over labeling legislation.

Lack of education regarding healthy food choices is a detriment to public health and safety — and *your* health and safety — and only stands to support the financial and political welfare of the GM seed manufacturers. Educating yourself by reading this and other reliable sources of GMO information is a good initial step towards making an informed choice to avoid or consume GMOs. With knowledge you can choose to support or not support GMO political endeavors.

22. WHAT ARE THE FDA FOOD LABELING GUIDELINES FOR GMOs?

In the U.S., many guidelines must be followed regarding the labeling of food products. Food labeling is required for most prepared foods, including canned and frozen foods, desserts, breads, cereals, and others. Nutrition labeling is also required for produce, but is voluntary for fish. Dietary supplements follow different labeling guidelines.

Labeling of GMOs in the U.S. is quite different from the labeling of most foods. The FDA requires GMOs to be labeled only in a few circumstances:

- if the food has a nutritional property significantly different from the organic food;
- if a new food contains any allergen that a consumer would not expect to be present; or
- if a food contains a toxin that is beyond acceptable limits.

In 2001, the FDA proposed voluntary guidelines for labeling GMOs and GM-free foods. These guidelines included using wording such as "GMO free," "Not genetically modified," "Genetically engineered," "This product contains high oleic acid soybean oil from soybeans developed using biotechnology to decrease the amount of saturated fat" or "The oil is made from soybeans that were not genetically engineered." Although the FDA has proposed only voluntary guidelines, there are many arguments by consumers over whether labeling of GM products should be mandatory.

23. HOW CAN ONE TELL IF THE FOODS THEY PURCHASE IN THE SUPERMARKET ARE GMO OR NOT? DOES "100% ORGANIC" MEAN NO GMO?

When a person picks a random item off a shelf in the grocery store, there is approximately a 70% chance that the random item contains genetically modified ingredients. Since Americans especially are largely uninformed about the prominence of GMOs on the market, many people do not realize they are purchasing GM products and are unaware of how to avoid such products. There are several ways to minimize one's chances of eating foods that have been genetically modified:

- **Buying foods that are "100% Organic"** is the easiest and best way to make sure that one's food contains no more than 0.01% GM ingredients. To be certified 100% organic, a food must be free from all GMOs, be produced with no artificial fertilizers or pesticides, and be taken from an animal reared without consistent use of antibiotics, growth hormones or other drugs.

  Although eating organic foods is the most effective way to avoid GMOs, GM crops are becoming more and more widespread. Because of this, wind pollination and the spread of GM seeds is causing even some organic products to be contaminated by GM elements. Organic farms are often located right next to non-organic farms that spray pesticides. Thus regulations allow a certain amount of pesticide residue on organic crops — it's unavoidable.

- **Reading labels carefully** is another way to avoid, at least in part, GM products. Be aware that the majority of all soybeans and corn products sold commercially in the U.S. have been genetically modified. Unless a product is specifically marked as organic, it is smart to keep an eye out for the following products known to contain GMOs:

malt and extract	food starch
sorbitol, dextrin	corn, malt syrup
confectioners' sugar	soybeans
Corn	rapeseed/canola
mayonnaise and other salad dressings that may contain lecithin	cottonseed oil (found in vegetable oil and margarine)
Zucchini	papayas
Miso	bread, pastry, baked goods

sugar beets	Dairy
chocolate, candy, chips, ice cream	sugar — GMO beet sugars are in many foods. Beet sugar that is GMO is marketed under the name "sugar." If the label says "cane sugar," there is some reassurance it is not GMO (but no guarantee).

- **Eat only 100% grass or pasture fed beef.** This same concept also applies to other herbivores like sheep. For poultry and pork, look for 100% organic, as these animals cannot be 100% grass fed.
- **Produce stickers** also help a consumer identify where their food is coming from, but some supermarkets may not use them. Specific codes indicate how a product was grown:
    - Four-digit codes, such as 1022, indicate conventionally grown
    - Five-digit codes beginning with 9, such as 91022, indicate organically grown
    - Five-digit codes beginning with 8, such as 81022, indicate genetically modified
- **Steering clear of processed foods,** which typically contain genetically modified ingredients, is also a smart idea. Speak with your local store manager and request the store implement a produce sticker system.
- **Shopping for locally-grown foods** can also reduce the risk of eating GMOs. Foods may be GMO-free if grown locally and not on industrial farms. Also, some seeds are still available that are GMO-free. Consider starting your own garden to grow fruits, vegetables and other foods.

Although it is becoming increasingly difficult to avoid GMOs, it is not impossible. Storeowners must be made aware that you want to know which foods are GMO and which are not. By not purchasing GMOs, you will send a message to the seed manufacturers that you do not want your foods genetically and unnaturally manipulated.

24. HOW DOES THE FDA CATEGORIZE FOOD ADDITIVES?

The FDA must premarket approve any food additives, defined as any substance added to a food product that has a significantly different structure, amount or function than other substances currently in the food. These additives must be approved whether or not they are products of genetic modification or biotechnology. The FDA uses recombinant DNA techniques to test whether a substance in food is an additive. However, if a product developed through genetic modification contains nothing significantly different from the original food, it is not required for that product to be premarket approved.

Products genetically engineered to contain pesticides or herbicides are also regulated by the EPA. The EPA's oversight seems to be missing the boat in its lack of awareness of the potential health risks of GMOs, evidenced by the fact that GMOs are all over the supermarket. What the FDA and EPA do not consider are the potential health dangers of combinations of individual chemicals that have been separately approved for human consumption. Even if the level of herbicides consumed by the average person is considered safe (*I take issue with this assumption*), there is no assurance that this is a "safe" amount of herbicide combined over a lifetime with other toxins in foods, drinks, the air and from other means.

Sadly, the environment inside and outside of our bodies has become more toxic than ever. These cumulative effects are known as bioaccumulation. When the body become overwhelmed with various toxins and cannot adequately detoxify them, health problems often result. Subtle or mysterious symptoms such as unexplained fatigue, memory issues, aches and pains, and chronic diseases such as inflammatory bowel diseases, cancers, diabetes, infertility and others may be, at least in part, the result of a lifetime of toxin accumulation. The concept of toxicity is not taken seriously in traditional medicine, except in extreme cases where the individual is exposed to toxicity at a work site. GMO manufacturers ignore the concept of bioaccumulation, leaving the public to fend for themselves. Thankfully, there are holistic or complementary health care providers with expertise in detoxification and health building.

25. WHAT IS INTELLECTUAL PROPERTY LAW AND HOW DOES IT RELATE TO GMOS?

Intellectual property refers to creations of the mind for which exclusive rights are given. These creations can include inventions, literary and artistic works, names, symbols and designs. Over the past decade, there has been considerable debate and controversy over the liabilities associated with GMOs. Legal issues have been raised in the production and use of GMO crops and the occurrence of contamination of GMO-free crops through transfer of seeds by wind or other means.

A farmer whose crops are contaminated by GM seed can face legal action for patent infringement if he replants his fields with seeds from contaminated plants. Companies that create GM crops have intellectual property rights, and have taken legal action against farmers who are unwitting victims of GM contamination. The court case *Monsanto v. Schmeiser* gives warning to farmers around the world to monitor their crops for the presence of GM seeds even if the farmers have no reason to believe that GM seed could potentially be present in their fields. Sadly, farmers are being sued out of existence unless they switch to purchasing GM seeds. The cross-contamination of crops, whether or not intentional, has seemingly motivated lawsuits to protect the GM seed monopoly, effectively driving out farmers who use non-GM seed.

How can the public trust an industry that would sue farmers for unintentional contamination of their non-GM crops with GM seeds? The lack of rectitude that would enable the GM seed industry to take such measures is deplorable. I question whether anything helpful to the population at large could arise from an industry that is more concerned about its own financial survival than the survival of the people.

26. HAVE THERE BEEN ANY EXAMPLES OF GMOS BEING DISCOVERED THAT WERE UNAPPROVED?

Unapproved GM wheat was recently found being grown in an Oregon field. This wheat posed a threat to trade with countries currently concerned about GMOs. Although the Agriculture Department came out with the statement that GM wheat is safe to consume and there is no evidence of the GM wheat entering the marketplace, the department is still skeptical about where the GM wheat came from. It is possible that the Oregon field was contaminated through wind pollination and that the farmers replanting the crop were unaware of the presence of GMOs. However, criminal wrongdoing is also being investigated.

As of now, the FDA has not approved genetically engineered wheat for U.S. farming. The wheat found in the Oregon field was of the same strain that was tested about a decade ago by Monsanto but never approved. The testing of the GM wheat was stopped in Oregon and several other states in 2005. Since Oregon exports approximately 90% of its wheat, this could be a potentially large problem. USDA officials have confirmed that no other incidences of GM wheat have been found.

This example of wheat contamination shows clearly that cross contamination cannot likely be completely controlled or avoided. Whether investigation determines improper conduct occurred, avoiding cross contamination of GMOs may be as impossible as guaranteeing a nuclear power plant near an earthquake fault will not have a meltdown. I do not think this comparison is extreme as the quality of one's health is in question in both instances and human error must always be factored in.

27. WHAT ARE ROUNDUP® READY CROPS AND HOW CAN THEY WITHSTAND EXPOSURE TO HIGHLY TOXIC ROUNDUP® HERBICIDES?

Crops that have been genetically engineered to withstand the herbicide *glyphosate*, the active ingredient in Monsanto's herbicide Roundup®, are known as Roundup® Ready (RR) crops. According to figures from the USDA, 94% of soybeans and approximately 70% of corn and cotton grown in the U.S. contain the Roundup® resistant gene. When planting glyphosate-tolerant crops, a farmer sprays the entire farm with glyphosate and can kill the weeds without harming the actual crop.

One concern with this herbicide is that its use will cause glyphosate-resistant weeds to grow. These weeds are sometimes referred to as "superweeds." Dow AgroScience created a strain of corn genetically engineered to withstand a different type of herbicide, 2, 4-D, a known carcinogen. New crops resistant to herbicide will be planted along organic crops. This causes the concern of cross contamination between the organic and genetically modified crops. As the herbicide is continuously used, more crops develop resistant genes. Several other concerns regarding the use of glyphosate should be considered before its production is genetically engineered into our food supply. (*Oops! Too late!*)

Consider several important points regarding glyphosate's potential harmful effects:

1. Toxicity is possible in humans with as little as >85 milliliters of concentrated glyphosate. Serious systemic and topical effects could include corrosive effects in the mouth and throat, epigastric pain (heartburn), unpleasant taste in the mouth, nasal discomfort, conjunctivitis, corneal injury, dysphagia (difficulty swallowing), liver and kidney impairment, respiratory distress, pulmonary edema, impaired consciousness, chest infiltration, heart arrhythmias (including ventricular present prior to death), metabolic acidosis, high blood calcium levels (hyperkalaemia) and even death.

2. Glyphosate works by inhibiting several plant enzymes including those needed to produce the amino acids phenylalanine, tryptophan and tyrosine in actively growing plants.

3. Glyphosate is also known to affect animal enzyme systems.

4. Glyphosate is toxic enough for the Environmental Protection Agency (EPA) to require products containing the glyphosate herbicide to carry a label warning against swallowing, urging the use of protective clothing when exposed to glyphosate, and instructing users not to go back into fields sprayed with glyphosate for at least four hours. Although glyphosate does not bio-accumulate in humans, meaning that it enters the body and then is excreted in the feces and urine, it still carries potential serious health risks, including death. The effects on the digestive and immune systems are only partly known.

5. No studies have examined the effects of glyphosate on our healthy gut flora required in part to regulate digestion, immunity and inflammation in the body.

6. Glyphosate is known to affect the bacterial ecology of the soil it is sprayed on and also causes micronutrient deficiencies in plants. Remember, we eat the plants with compromised micronutrient levels.

7. Glyphosate may contain various "inert" compounds or adjuvants that are unknown to us because U.S. federal regulations do not insist on full disclosure of inert materials.

GMO proponents downplay these potential dangers, declaring the amount of glyphosate that reaches the individual consumer is far too insignificant. It is important to note the EPA caught Monsanto scientists who were studying glyphosate falsifying test results on two separate occasions. The first incident involved Biotest Laboratories (IBT), resulting in the closing of this lab by the U.S. Justice Department in 1978. Higher-ups at IBT Labs were found guilty of falsifying statements and scientific data they had submitted to the government for review. The second incident in 1991 involved Don Cravan, owner of Cravan Laboratories, and three employees. The employees were indicted on 20 felony counts and Mr. Cravan, with 14 additional employees, were found guilty and punished on similar charges.

28. WHAT IS BT CORN AND HOW IS IT GENETICALLY ENGINEERED?

Bt corn is a genetically modified crop. Like any other GMO, the genetic trait of interest in a plant is identified and then separated from the rest of the genetic material in the donor organism. The donor organism can be a fungus, another plant or a bacterium. The donor organism used to produce Bt corn is called Bacillus thuringiensis, a soil bacterium containing a protein that is effective in killing caterpillar larvae, which are a nuisance to farmers and their corn crops. The protein, Bt delta endotoxin, is inserted into the corn crops to reproduce as an alternative to spraying insecticides.

In essence, corn has become an herbicide factory! What is worse, pro-GMO manufacturers claim BT is entirely safe and do not seem to understand why intelligent people would not want to eat Bt pesticide. An educated public would not blindly trust Bt corn from a company that has a history of misleading and fraudulent claims – especially when long-term human studies have not been conducted to date. Common sense should tell us that consuming pesticides is dangerous for one's health. Safe exposure to the Bt toxin cannot be fully studied, as individuals will have varying tolerance to Bt toxin in the short- and long-run. It is simply not possible to determine how many cases of cancer, neurologic disorders, autoimmune diseases, intestinal issues and other health problems increasingly experienced by the American public are the result of years of Bt toxin consumption.

29. HOW DOES THE INSECTICIDE BT THAT HAS BEEN DIRECTLY INSERTED INTO CORN KILL INSECTS THAT FEED ON THE CORN?

Bacillus thuringiensis (Bt) is soil-dwelling bacterium, commonly used as a biological pesticide. Bt is used to make a GM insecticide gene that is inserted into plants such as corn in order to produce crops that can protect themselves from insects. By using Bt crops, farmers do not need to spray additional insecticides to kill specific harmful insects. In Europe, Bt corn produces a protein called Bt delta endotoxin, which kills Lepidoptera larvae, or caterpillars, and more specifically, the European corn borer.

Bt delta endotoxin was selected for use because it is extremely efficient at protecting crops from Lepidoptera during the larval stage, the most harmful stage. A plant with Bt contains the Bt protein in only part of the plant. A susceptible insect must ingest the part of the plant containing the Bt. Once ingested, the protein immediately binds to the wall of the gut in the insect, causing the insect to stop feeding. Within a few hours, the wall of the gut breaks down entirely and the body cavity becomes invaded with normal gut bacteria. As the bacteria multiply in the insect's bloodstream, the insect dies of septicaemia. Though the protein is very effective, even among caterpillar larvae species have differing sensitivities to the protein, so 100% of the insects aren't always killed.

The Bt protein was also chosen because of its apparent safety. Since the protein is claimed to be selective, insects that do not feed on corn such as beetles or ladybugs are not harmed (so it's claimed). The Bt protein is also considered safe for humans as well as other mammals, and other parts of the ecosystem and environment.

I have a few issues with the claims that Bt is safe for humans and the environment. First, even if the Bt protein is selective against insects that eat corn, killing off these insects would create an unnatural ratio of corn-eating insects to non-corn eating insects. The environment as a whole depends upon a balanced ecosystem. It is reasonable to expect that the insect populations would adjust to a change in even one species of insect. A change in the insect population may affect the population of birds that feed on the remaining insects. Bird and insect population adjustments may promote changes in the surrounding forestry. These and other unforeseen ecological changes could have profound effects upon the local and distant environments. Adverse and unnatural changes in the environment can and often do have a ripple effect upon both human health and the natural order of ecological systems.

30. HOW DOES BT FUNCTION AS AN INSECTICIDE FOR CROP CONTROL? IS THERE A LINK BETWEEN BT AND COLONY COLLAPSE DISORDER?

Bt (Bacillus thuringiensis) insecticides are most commonly used to prevent against insects such as leaf-eating caterpillars that feed on and kill crops. Bt's unusual properties enable it to infect and kill insects that eat the GM plant containing. Bt produces proteins that attach to the gut lining of specific insects and paralyze the digestive system to stop the insect from feeding. After several days, the insect dies from starvation. For some insects, the Bt proteins enter the insect and multiply until the Bt attains the desired effect. For other insects, the Bt proteins are immediately lethal and do not have to multiply before killing the insect.

Colony Collapse Disorder (CCD) refers to an entire beehive or bee colony dying off. A study done by Hans-Hinrich Kaatz found that bee colonies fed Bt contained a significant reduction in the number of broods in the Bt colony as compared to a colony fed Bt toxin-free pollen. There were a reduced number of broods in both colonies, though the Bt-fed bees had a greater reduction. This shows that Bt is certainly a potential factor for the colony collapse phenomenon. Other CCD findings showed that bees in contact with Bt had sting glands scarred with black marks. This type of darkening on the sting gland indicates an immune response to a harmful pathogen. The bees that were not in contact with the Bt did not show such marks. Researchers are still studying the possible link between Bt and CCD.

The nightmarish consequences of tampering with nature through GMOs continue to unfold, as one of the worst fears associated with them are being seen — honeybees are dying off at an alarming rate around the globe. While some adverse effects of GMOs manifest quickly, the reduction in the bee population is one of the more insidious ones, manifesting somewhat more slowly. In 2006 beekeepers started to notice sharp declines in their honeybee (Apis melifera) colonies. Seasonal declines in honeybee colonies are normal, but the severity and persistence of the decline observed first by beekeepers along the east coast of the U.S. prompted scientists to delineate this phenomenon as CCD. Most reports indicate that most beekeepers in the U.S. have experienced as much as a 30% reduction on average from winter to winter.

There is no general consensus among scientists as to what is causing CCD, but scientists agree the agricultural, economic and environmental impact of this problem will be devastating to global environmental stability in complex ways. Honeybees are absolutely essential for pollination of U.S. agriculture. Honeybees are the most economically valuable type of bee for agricultural pollination of crops worldwide and in the United States. In the U.S., bee pollination of crops accounts for approximately one-third of the U.S. diet in the form of fruits, vegetables, forage crops, tree nuts, certain field crops and other specialty crops.

The monetary value of honeybees as pollinators for commercial crops throughout the U.S. exceeds $15 billion annually and may be as high as $20 billion. CCD has resulted in substantial loss of crops from reduced total yields (production) and quality of produced crops. CCD has also affected seed production. Alfalfa production in the form mostly of alfalfa hay has been significantly affected by the reduction in honey bee pollination. Apples, citrus, cotton, almonds and soybean production has also been adversely affected. GM crops may be adversely affecting honeybees not dissimilarly to how they are known to affect certain other insects such as moths and caterpillars. I believe that there are simply too many unanswered questions regarding the toxic impact of GMOs on humans, other mammals and certain insects…including possibly the honeybee.

The connection between Colony Collapse Disorder being observed currently and GMOs cannot be ignored. I believe that there is a connection between the declining population of honeybees and the introduction into the environment of transgenic foods and in particular Bt corn. Bt corn has been genetically modified to express the Cry1Ab protein of *Bacillus thuringiensis* to kill lepidopteran pests. Thus, Bt corn produces, as a result of its genetic modification, herbicide that can be toxic to many varieties of insects including honeybees, not to mention to the environment as a whole and all species of mammals.

31. ACCORDING TO THE GREENSHARE *FACTSHEETS*, WHAT ARE THE DISADVANTAGES OF THE BT TOXIN?

According to GreenShare, there are four main disadvantages of using Bt toxin in transgenic crops:

1. Bt is susceptible to degrading in the sunlight. This degradation can occur less than a week following application of the Bt. Newer strains of Bt developed to control leaf beetles, for example, have become ineffective in fewer than 24 hours.

2. Bt is a highly specific toxin, which may cause crops to be destroyed by other insects that the Bt does not account for, including aphids or grasshoppers.

3. Bt may prove ineffective when eaten by a target insect if the Bt is not applied thoroughly to the plant. Insects that tunnel into plants, including the earthworm, may never come in contact with any part of the plant containing the Bt.

4. Bt products tend to have shorter shelf lives than other pesticides by approximately two to three years of storage.

STUDY SUMMARY:

"Bacillus thuringiensis (Bt) Transgenic Crop: An Environment Friendly Insect-Pest Management Strategy"

According to this paper, Bt provides an effective alternative to DDT, a poisonous chemical insecticide that had adverse environmental effects. Bt saves both money and time, reduces health risks and has a safe history. There is concern regarding the resistance of insects to one or more Cry proteins. However, the "high-dose/refuge strategy" has proven most promising in approach to prolonging the effectiveness of Bt toxins. Although there are many ethical and moral issues regarding genetically modified organisms, especially Bt, Bt crops are rapidly increasing globally. More than 32 million acres have been cultivated worldwide.

Author's note: In contrast to this article, I have cited throughout this book many potential adverse effects of Bt insecticide upon human health, other mammals, insects and the environment.

32. WHAT DID THE NOVEMBER 1999 ARTICLE ON GMO SAFETY IN THE *LANCET*, A LEADING BRITISH MEDICAL JOURNAL, SHOW REGARDING THE EFFECT OF GMO CONSUMPTION ON EXPERIMENTAL ANIMALS?

This study aimed to observe the effects of GM potato diets on the transformation of rat guts. The scientists found there was an increase in intestinal crypt cell proliferation rate and crypt size in the gut of the rat. Increased cellular proliferation is a hallmark of inflammatory damage and cancer. Intestinal infections were found in the rats as well. The study has been questioned by other researchers as to how well it was performed. Pusztai and the other scientists who originally performed the study have been willing to re-conduct it, though they assure the public their study was performed in a professional manor. The study suggests that it is not safe for mammals to consume GM products, specifically GM potatoes, which were seen to have drastic and damaging effects on the mammalian gut. Such effects would have no other cause but from the GMO.

33. WHAT DID ONE OF THE EDITORS OF THE *LANCET* CLAIM REGARDING PUBLISHING CONTROVERSIAL RESEARCH QUESTIONING THE SAFETY OF GMOS?

In a 1999 article published by the British newspaper, the *Guardian*, Richard Horton, editor of the *Lancet*, claims he was threatened in a phone call from an officer of the Royal Society if he published Pusztai's controversial research regarding GM food safety. The *Guardian* determined the caller to be Peter Lachmann, the former vice president of the Royal Society and president of the Academy of Medical Sciences, an advocate of GMOs. Lachmann believes GMOs can help hunger, prevent disease and have many other benefits. He reportedly accused Horton over the phone of knowing Dr. Pusztai's study results to be "untrue." Lachmann also implied that publishing Pusztai's paper in the *Lancet* would have consequences for Horton's career as an editor.

Lachmann denied making any inappropriate or threatening remarks toward Horton, stating instead that he warned Horton of making the mistake of publishing a paper with results that were in need of further research. Lachmann termed Pusztai's study "bad science." In March, the Royal Society decided to scrutinize Pusztai's study and found that the data appeared to be "flawed in many aspects." The *Guardian*, however, established that the Royal Society was attempting to prevent Pusztai's paper from ever being published, as the public would be offered an opinion that demonstrated the negative consequences of consuming GM products.

COMMENT: THE ROLE OF THE MEDIA

A few words about mainstream media are warranted. Over my 25 years of clinical practice I have written hundreds of articles for both professional periodicals and the lay public. I have also appeared on numerous television and radio shows and have learned a few things from these experiences about how to expertly serve as a professional information source. The media's job is to make news. I once asked a former producer for Fox Five News, why he didn't report on happier stories instead of all of the doom-and-gloom that so pervades our media. He said, "We provide the type of stories that the public wants," to which I responded, "How do you know that they don't want happier stories"? He had no response, and from the look on his face I could tell he had no proof of what the public wanted or needed. My point is this: if the public makes enough noise, the media will take notice and often side with the majority opinion. This is not always true, of course, but it does clearly demonstrate that if the public wants Frankenfood dangers exposed, the media must take notice, become educated and report their stories from a balanced, unbiased perspective.

People involved in media — television, newspapers and other print and online periodicals — often know very little about their subject topic. They are provided with an assignment and use various websites and outlets to locate "qualified" professionals to make their point. And so the media-machine trudges on spewing out story after story to attract attention and ultimately to gather paid advertisers. Sadly, the "tone" of a topic of interest is almost entirely determined by the media, which is composed of individuals who are mostly "just doing their jobs" and are often not uniquely trained to sufficiently investigate a story topic. Hopefully books like this one will help cut through the morass of ignorance that pervades the media surrounding the GMO topic so that the public's inherent right to be informed is maintained and not trampled upon by special interest groups.

FOX News Interview

In 2013, I was invited to FOX News studios for an interview, head-to-head with geneticists from Cornell University, on the topic of GMOs. I was told that questions would be posed to both me and the geneticists. I arrived at the studio and was politely greeted and escorted onto the interview set. As I sat in the chair across from my interviewer, she received a text message from the geneticists she was scheduled to interview in just a few minutes. My interviewer said that the geneticists had concerns about a live interview with me and insisted on a separate interview, after my interview, to directly answer her questions and presumably my responses. In effect, they wanted the last word and to have time to prepare responses. I was prepared for the questions and had anticipated responding to the same misleading statements that geneticists and other pro-GMO advocates typically would rely on — statements like, "GMOs are exactly the same as non-GMOs produced by 'natural selection.'" Another common statement by pro-GMO folks is that GMOs have been studied and proven not to pose health problems. My responses would have been short and to the point: "GMOs are produced by entirely artificial processes using a gene gun, and insert traits in plants that would not occur though natural selection, such as the insertion of strawberry genes into salmon. Regarding safety studies, not enough have been done and the question of safety is very real." My professional opinion as a natural health care provider is to avoid Frankenfoods at all costs...and keep your health!

The refusal of pro-GMO representatives to participate in rational interviews on national television is nothing new. On an episode of the Dr. Oz show, I was astounded to see how the producers of the show allowed pro-GMO folks to refuse to take the same stage as anti-GMO proponents. Dr. Oz announced that this would occur at the very start of the show, but did not reveal the obvious truth, in my opinion, of this tactic — namely, that Dr. Oz and his producers likely folded under the pressure and insistence of the pro-GMO representatives because they felt that they could not provide an adequate defense for the well-prepared pro-health, anti-GMO experts. This is what I believe happened; what other explanation could there be? This tactic of pro-GMO representatives attempting to get the upper hand always fails and suggests deceit and manipulation. Thankfully, the public is becoming too smart and is not so easily fooled by such tactics. The evidence is the growing awareness of the GMO controversy.

The geneticists interviewed seemed nice and provided information that sounded reasonable on the surface. But much of what was said represents many misunderstandings on the part of the geneticists. Bottom line: to understand GMO issues, every one of us must spend some time sifting through the truths, half-truths and misunderstandings that are perpetuated in the media. A portion of my interview can be found on the Fox News website at http://fxn.ws/12NmSBJ.

34. WHAT IS THE FRENCH STUDY THAT DEMONSTRATED FEEDING GMOS TO ANIMALS PRODUCED TUMORS?

Researchers from the Committee for Research & Independent Information on Genetic Engineering (CRIIGEN) reported in *Food and Chemical Toxicology* on the results of an alarming two-year study using rats. In the study, headed by Gilles-Eric Seralini of the University of Caen, rats were fed either NK603 Roundup-tolerant genetically modified maize cultivated with and without Roundup®, and Roundup® alone, at the levels at which the U.S. permits in GM crops and drinking water.

No Testing of GMOs or GM Pesticides

Currently, the U.S. does not require any sort of mandatory animal testing for GMOs or GM pesticides. The 90-day study using feeding trials revealed shocking and unprecedented data confirming the cancer-causing effects of GMOs and agricultural chemicals. For all three treated groups, two to three times more female rats died than in the control group, and more rapidly. The study noted:

> This difference was visible in 3 male groups fed GMOs. All results were hormone and sex dependent, and the pathological profiles were comparable. Females developed large mammary tumors almost always more often than and before controls, the pituitary was the second most disabled organ; the sex hormonal balance was modified by GMO and Roundup® treatments. In treated males, liver congestions and necrosis were 2.5–5.5 times higher. This pathology was confirmed by optic and transmission electron microscopy. Marked and severe kidney nephropathies were also generally 1.3–2.3 greater. Males presented 4 times more large palpable tumors than controls, which occurred up to 600 days earlier. Biochemistry data confirmed very significant kidney chronic deficiencies; for all treatments and both sexes, 76% of the altered parameters were kidney related. These results can be explained by the non-linear endocrine-disrupting effects of Roundup®, but also by the overexpression of the transgene in the GMO and its metabolic consequences.

The results of the study are extremely disconcerting. The study confirmed that the levels of GM chemicals currently allowed in foods and agricultural pesticides in the U.S. and many other countries are scientifically proven to cause tumors. Increased cancer in the population can also be linked to the findings of this study. Critics who oppose anti-GMO efforts consistently point out the faults of studies that suggest GMO dangers. In my view, scientific studies are fraught with bias and poor design, and are often undermined by financial interests. Practically any scientific study can be criticized for having a poor design, incorrect conclusions, and for other reasons deemed a fraud. Truly independent study is nearly impossible and studies are often inherently biased with the researchers' obvious or hidden agendas. The scientific community itself has questioned the integrity of the double-blind placebo controlled study in reflecting real-life outcomes. It is important for the layperson and scientist to remember that scientific studies are not real life and any conclusions drawn from them must be considered very carefully.

Studies performed on animals may not apply to humans. Furthermore, many studies are based on "average" people. I have never met an "average" person, and scientific studies are based on grouping many people together for average conclusions.

Bottom line: The findings of the French Study should not be ignored, but by the same token should not be considered as the "final say" in terms of accuracy. Rather than only pointing out the possible design flaws of this study, those who criticize it should volunteer constructive suggestions leading towards cooperation that ultimately results in making the best possible decisions for public safety. Proper study should be performed *before* GMOs, or any other major factor, are unleashed into the human food chain and environment.

STUDY SUMMARY:

"Safety and Nutritional Assessment of GM Plants and Derived Food and Feed: The Role of Animal Feeding Trials"

This study discusses the elements of an assessment procedure for GM food and feed. The study also discusses the aspect of animal trials to ensure safety of GM products, and how animal studies can have both potential and limitations. In assessing the safety of a GM product, both regular GM and nutritionally enhanced GM products are studied. A safety assessment compares GM food and feed to their conventional counterparts. In determining how a GM product varies in biological structure to its counterpart, a comparative phenotype and molecular analysis of the new product is carried out. Significant differences of the GM analysis to the conventional food would indicate unintentional but possibly harmful effects of the GMO, and the product would be tested further.

Many animal studies have been performed to assess the safety of GM products when ingested. However, many of these studies do not indicate clinical effects of the food or histopathological abnormalities in the tissues or organs of the animals that ingested the GMO. Studies have also assessed the performance potential of livestock that consume GM feed versus non-GM feed.

To test whole food and feed, 90-day rodent studies have been deemed appropriate for assessing food safety. The purpose of this type of study is to determine potential effects of toxins or nutritional components in the whole food. The study considers the characteristics of new traits that result from the nature of the food or feed as compared to their intended role. Ninety-day studies appear long enough to determine whether adverse effects appear as a result of chemicals in the GM product.

Author's note: In my judgment, tests and procedures available at present, including those reviewed in this paper, are certainly not perfect and occasionally result in false-positive and false-negative results. Until more accurate assessments to detect the presence of GMOs are developed, these Frankenfoods should not be released into our diets or the environment.

35. WHAT ARE THE CRITICISMS OF THE FRENCH STUDY AND THE EFFECTS OF GMOS ON RATS?

The two-year French study that appeared in *Food and Chemical Toxicology* prompted high concern and criticism of GMOs, specifically Monsanto's genetically modified corn. Rats were shown to develop large tumors and multiple organ damage when fed GMO corn sprayed with Roundup® weed killer. However, experts not involved in the study are skeptical of the findings. Tom Sanders, head of the nutritional sciences research division at King's College London, pointed out that Seralini and his team of researchers failed to report in their findings how much they had given the rats to eat or what the growth rates of the rats were. "This strain of rat is very prone to mammary tumors particularly when food intake is not restricted," Sanders noted. "The statistical methods are unconventional."

Mark Tester, a research professor at the Australian Centre for Plant Functional Genomics at the University of Adelaide, wondered why the extreme findings of this study had not been noted in any previous studies with Monsanto GMOs. Tester questioned, "If the effects are as big as purported, and if the work really is relevant to humans, why aren't the North Americans dropping like flies? GMOs have been in the food chain for over a decade over there — and longevity continues to increase inexorably." David Spiegelhalter of the University of Cambridge pointed out how the methods, statistics and reporting of the results of the study were below standard. He also noted how the control group used in the study was comprised of 10 female and 10 male rats, most of which also developed tumors.

Mr. Tester probably means well, but what makes him think we in North America are not dropping like flies? He clearly has a limited concept of how GM food consumption could affect the population over the long-term and how a decreasing quality of life is on the rise – this is what I have observed first hand over the last 25 years as a health care provider. Continued environmental exposure of humans to various toxins is a fact and is occurring right now. It is practically impossible to conduct long-term studies on the health effects on humans given our long lifespans. Systemic diseases such as cancer and immune diseases including multiple sclerosis, Hashimoto's hypothyroidism, lupus, Sjogren's syndrome, diabetes and others occur over many years, making cause-and-effect almost impossible to determine.

Although the French study has faults, virtually any scientific study can be criticized. Science is not perfect. In fact, the entire "scientific method" itself has been called into question as a valid research technique. Having said this, more studies should be done, but by truly independent groups that are focused on the long- and short-term health effects upon humans, insects, farm animals and the environment. Modern day physicians' skills are best at discerning acute illness, the type that happens right away and affects the population at large. Those skills fail miserably when it comes to disease recognition and prevention in the long term. Certain cancers, inflammatory bowel disease, special needs issues and autoimmune diseases are on the rise since the introduction of GMOs in the U.S. Could this association between greater GMO consumption by Americans and disease be coincidental? Yes, but coincidence should not be assumed. As for the reasons why other studies have not obtained the same findings as the French study — that's easy! Bias and hidden agendas on the part of GMO seed manufacturers would account for both the lack of study and findings of any potential health risks.

COMMENT: THERE IS LITTLE SCIENCE IN GMO SCIENTIFIC STUDIES

A few words regarding the fallibility of the scientific method are in order. I am not sure, given current scientific methods, if the potential dangers of GMOs can ever be fully tested or appreciated. Sometimes one must rely on "common sense." The problem with common sense in politics, society and the scientific community is that common sense is not at all common. As a holistic doctor, I see and think about the world from a natural perspective. I superimpose in my thoughts on issues such as GMOs within a mental and intellectual framework of "natural," "do no harm" and "how would nature work here." This perspective is, I freely admit, my bias. Pro-GMO doctors, scientists and uneducated individuals think in terms of scientific methods and often renounce nature. No wonder there is such controversy over the GMO issue. Ultimately, bias is inherent within all human endeavors –

including politics and science. What should remain as a fundamental tenet of honest assessment is public safety and sincere integrity, so that health and safety choices can be made in the interest of quality of life improvement and not for political and ultimately financial reasons.

36. WHAT ARE EXAMPLES OF COMMERCIALLY AVAILABLE BIOTECH CROPS THAT HAVE PRESUMABLY BEEN STUDIED FOR SAFETY?

All biotech crops on the market must be approved for their equivalence to their conventional food counterparts, their nutritional value and the possible implications. Although the U.S. does not currently require labeling on all GM products, those being commercially sold have been approved for safety by properly performed scientific methods. Many crops are available commercially that use biotech seeds, including sweet corn, field corn, soybeans, cotton, canola, rapeseed, sugar beets, papayas, alfalfa and squash. These Frankenfoods have shown to cause health problems that, in my view, support their immediate removal from agriculture.

37. WHICH GMOS ARE FED TO LIVESTOCK SUCH AS COWS, CHICKENS AND PIGS, AND DO THEY POSE A HEALTH RISK?

In the last 50 years, the way animals are fed has changed dramatically. Animals are fed with little consideration to what is best for the animals or for human health. Common ingredients in livestock feed include scraps of same species meat (sometimes from diseased animals), feathers, hair, skin, hooves, blood, manure and other animal waste, plastics, drugs and chemicals, and unhealthy amounts of grains. Now, thanks to the GMO seed manufacturers and various governmental agencies, GMOs have been added to our food supply, adding to the "toxic stew" of daily food choices.

The feed given to livestock is largely genetically modified. Especially in Europe, cows, pigs and chickens are eating GMOs. Feed for these animals usually contain ingredients from GM plants. GM animal feed is required to be labeled, but the milk, eggs and meat taken from the livestock does not require labeling. Soy and soy meat, the most popular and inexpensive ingredient in livestock feed, is largely genetically modified. Of the 40 million tons of raw soy product annually imported into Europe, half of that product goes to livestock feed.

Another common ingredient in livestock feed is corn. Corn is also widely genetically modified, even more so than we can measure due to the wind pollination that carries genetically modified seed to corn crops in other countries. Feed additives are also genetically engineered. Various additives and enzymes added to livestock feed are produced with the help of genetically modified microorganisms. Some additives in feed are so toxic that they are removed from the diet of livestock before their slaughter. Some examples of additives to which livestock may be exposed include larvacides and various medications, including potentially cancer-causing antibiotics and growth hormones. Many medications are routinely used in livestock to control acidosis, improve feeding habits of confined animals, promote increased wait gain, prevent coccidiosis (a parasitic disease), treat/prevent bacterial enteritis from E. coli bacterial infection, prevent bacterial diarrhea and treat shipping fever in cattle. Residues of medications are found with the foods eaten by most Americans each and every day. Now, we can add GMOs to the list of foods that I fear will continue to tip the health-disease balance towards disease. The potentially devastating health effects of Frankenfoods on humans may be compounded by the concentration of GMO products that are fed to the livestock many Americans consume.

38. WHAT IS RECOMBINANT BOVINE SOMATOTROPIN (rBST)? WHAT IS POSILAC? WHAT EFFECT DOES rBST HAVE ON COWS' PRODUCTION OF MILK?

The synthetic protein hormone rBST, used mainly by dairy farmers to increase the production of milk in cows, was approved by the FDA on November 5, 1993. Bovine somatotropin (BST) is the natural form of growth hormone in cattle; rBST refers to BST that has been genetically engineered in a lab. The hormone stimulates the milk production of cattle by increasing the levels of IGF1, or a hormone known as insulin-like growth factor.

Posilac, Monsanto's version of rBST, is used by farmers to increase a cow's milk production. Posilac is applied to the cow's udder approximately 50 days into the cow's lactation. Posilac works by sustaining the mammary cells and limiting the rate of decrease of milk production after production peaks. The FDA determined BST safe for human health. However, public concern about BST relates to the fact that the form of BST given to cows is recombinant — derived from yeast or bacteria with the BST gene from cattle — that has been inserted into their genome or genetic material. Studies exist that suggest large or inappropriate exposure to BST-like proteins is dangerous to human beings and other animals.

39. WHAT IS THE CONTROVERSY REGARDING rBST AND HUMAN HEALTH?

There is much controversy regarding rBST and its effect on human health. No biological side effects have been seen in humans who ingest the rBST present in cow's milk; however, there have been some side effects for the cattle injected with rBST. One of these side effects includes an increased risk of mastitis, a type of udder infection. Several groups of consumers and researchers have expressed concern over the safety of ingesting any milk containing rBST. It is likely that rBST can make its way into the human body as a direct result of cow's milk consumption. If the proves to be true, a variety of health problems can result in humans, including cancer, infertility, mastitis and others.

Traces of antibiotics or penicillin-based drugs used to treat mastitis in cattle may be found in cow's milk. There are fears that such drugs in the milk could cause allergic reactions and an increase in IGF1 in humans. IGF1 also stimulates growth of intestinal cells, leading to abnormal intestinal growth. Consumers fear that IGF1 in milk may be carcinogenic to humans. In summary, livestock are fed and stuffed with dozens of medications, chemicals, foods of poor quality and potentially GMO, and are placed under tremendous stress. If you choose to eat these foods, you should not expect to maximize your health potential.

40. WHAT DOES MONSANTO SAY ABOUT MILK PROCESSORS THAT HAVE CHOSEN TO LABEL THEIR MILK rBST FREE?

Many farmers have expressed concerns about the safety of using rBST on their cattle and have opted to label their products with "From cows not treated with rBST." In 1994, the FDA said that such a label statement was acceptable. However, in early 2007, Monsanto appealed to the FDA and FTC to declare that such labels are misleading. The FTC replied to Monsanto's appeal with the statement, "The FTC staff agrees with FDA that food companies may inform consumers in advertising, as in labeling, that they do not use rBST." Though Monsanto and its endorsers believe that the public should not have the right to know if rBST is in their food, as of now, consumers still have such a right.

41. WHAT DOES MONSANTO CLAIM IS THEIR ROLE IN FOOD PRODUCTION?

Monsanto claims its primary role in food production is to produce genetically modified seeds. Monsanto produces a great variety of seeds, both conventional and genetically modified, for products that can be grown in many different areas of the world. Monsanto is an agricultural company that claims to grow high-quality crops that contribute to a safe, healthful and sustainable food supply. They do this by selling seeds to farmers who can provide a wide variety of products for consumers to buy.

Monsanto claims to be committed to sharing all information about safety and benefits of their seeds and the products that they produce. Monsanto labels all of their seed products to ensure that farmers know what they are buying, though not all consumers are aware of what they are buying because labeling is not required on most GM products.

Monsanto also alleges safety is their number one priority, and that they work with many researchers, health societies and scientists to learn more about the products they are creating via genetic engineering. They claim to use the results of studies and research to make sure that genetically engineered crops are just as safe as their conventional counterparts. Their claims of equivalent safety of GM versus non-GM products do not appear to be true, however. I have cited many examples throughout this book describing nutritional deficiencies, potential allergies, serious intestinal problems and other health issues that fly in the face of Monsanto's safety claims.

During an interview where I appeared on FOX News, a geneticist claimed GMOs have shown no health hazards in humans in the 15 years they have been available to consumers. This geneticist and others seem unwilling to consider GMO consumption could have contributed at least in part to the rise of various cancers, autoimmune diseases or food-borne illnesses, which have been primarily attributed to bacterial, yeast and parasitic contamination...why not GMO contamination?

42. HOW MANY FARMERS IN THE U.S. GROW GMO PRODUCTS?

As of 2012, 17.3 million farmers grew GM crops. This record-breaking number is up from 16.7 million in 2011. Since 1996, 173 million GM crops were planted in 28 countries, a 100-fold increase in GM production.

43. IS THERE ANY EVIDENCE THAT GM PRODUCTION DECREASES RATHER THAN INCREASES FOOD YIELD?

Though many endorsers of GM crops believe that such crops increase food yield, there is also evidence suggesting GM products actually decrease food yield in the U.S. and throughout the world. The process of genetic modification of foods has caused a 50% drop in food production. Field tests performed on Bt corn have shown that corn containing the toxin takes longer than conventional corn to reach maturity. GM corn has produced up to 12% lower yields than non-GM corn.

Monsanto's claim that genetic modification is the solution to having higher yields has been disputed in many reports. In a report authored by Doug Gurian-Sherman, former EPA scientist, he stated in his peer-reviewed studies that GM herbicide resistant soybeans and GM herbicide resistant corn have not increased in their yields. The report also noted that since the year 2000, yield increases in both crops came almost entirely from traditional breeding of the product and not from genetic modification.

44. WHAT MEASURES SHOULD BE TAKEN TO INSURE THE SAFETY OF PROTEINS INTRODUCED INTO THE FOOD CHAIN THROUGH GENETIC MODIFICATION?

One process used to judge the safety of genetically engineered foods is the substantial equivalence concept. This process shows the degree to which a genetically modified plant or animal differs from its conventional counterpart and also helps to identify any increased health hazards that may be found in the new food. Various tests are used to identify the degree of substantial equivalence, including the testing of chemical composition, levels of toxins, nutritional quality, and more. If notable differences are found between the genetically modified food and its counterpart, then the food must be examined further to ensure its safety for human consumption.

All genetically modified foods currently on the market have been approved by these safety tests. However, as biotechnological practices in foods become more complex, judging the safety of foods becomes increasingly difficult. Progress must be made in identifying proteins found in genetically modified foods that may be potential allergens.

45. WHAT IS THE ILSI CROP COMPOSITION DATABASE?

The ILSI Crop Composition database was created as a project by the International Life Sciences Institute (ILSI). The project represents a coalescence of crop analyses from various agricultural companies. The participants in the project have pooled data about their crops, both conventional and genetically engineered, to make such data available to the general public, government agencies and industry. Version 4 was released in 2010; different versions of the project are constantly being worked on. More information regarding the ILSI database can be found at their website, www.cropcomposition.org.

46. ACCORDING TO MONSANTO, WHAT ARE THE KEY COMPONENTS OF THE FOOD/FEED SAFETY ASSESSMENT?

Monsanto assesses the safety of genetically modified food or feed by first comparing the GMO to the conventional food it was derived from. The ILSI Crop Composition database is an important resource to help judge whether biologically important changes have occurred in the composition of the GM food or feed. The ILSI is also an important research tool for assessing nutritionally enhanced crops, as a significant change in composition is intentional. To determine the safety and nutritional value of biotech crops, each food must be assessed individually, and in some cases, studies involving rats are conducted to provide additional assurance of safety.

47. IN ADDITION TO THE NUTRITIONAL COMPARISONS INVOLVED IN COMPARATIVE STUDIES OF GMO AND NON-GMO COUNTERPARTS, WHAT ELSE IS COMPARED?

Nutritional comparisons are the main form of assessing GMOs. Scientists also compare the amounts of vitamins and minerals found in GMOs. For example, GMO corn has 14 ppm of calcium, while its non-GM counterpart contains 6130 ppm. GMO corn also contains only 2 ppm of magnesium, while non-GM corn contains 113 ppm. Where is the "nutritional equivalence" in these examples? And, if nutritional equivalence is a myth, what myths might underlie other GMO claims? I think many of them we have and will continue to explore throughout this book.

Scientists also look to see what, if any, new toxins can be found in GMOs. Currently, the EPA allows for the amount of glyphosate in water in the U.S. to be 0.7ppm, although European tests have shown that animals develop organ damage at .0001 ppm. GMO corn contains 13 ppm of glyphosate, which is 130,000 times higher than the level deemed toxic in our water. GMO corn also contains 200 times the formaldehyde shown to be toxic to animals when ingested. Other comparisons made between GMOs and non-GMOs include the number of diseases they could cause, the number and expense of medical costs, the quality of manure, and whether the foods will lead to increased or decreased feed consumption.

48. WHAT INSECTICIDE RESISTANCE MANAGEMENT STRATEGIES FOR GM CROPS ARE BEING USED THROUGHOUT THE WORLD? WHAT CONTROVERSIES REVOLVE AROUND THESE STRATEGIES AND HOW ARE SUCH CONTROVERSIES BEING APPROACHED?

New plant-incorporated protectant crops (PIP) have been applied widely throughout the U.S., resulting in higher crop yields, lower need for other insecticides and control of mycotoxin content. Though the U.S. has approved these crops, Europe and many other countries have not. The Environmental Protection Agency's Office of Pesticide Programs has been analyzing the management of PIP crops and has instituted new regulations regarding Bt crops. To further develop sustainable insecticide resistant strategies, the EPA Office of Research and Development and the Office of Pesticide Programs will be working together to develop new solutions. I am personally against the use of any chemical sprayed or otherwise exposed to the foods that we consume.

49. DOES THE FACT THAT HUNDREDS OF MILLIONS OF MEALS CONTAIN GMOS MEAN THE FOODS ARE SAFE?

Monsanto declares that the ever-increasing consumption of GMOs by millions of people inherently implies safety. The consumption of Frankenfoods, in reality, implies underhanded politics that I believe have forwarded Monsanto's ultimate agenda: namely, to corner the food market and to circumvent public notification, education and awareness. It is virtually impossible to determine long-term health effects of GM products on the human body, as most studies on the safety of these products are done on a short-term basis and are never performed on humans. The impact of GMOs upon human health has not yet been carried out in rigorous, double-blind scientific studies. Monsanto has made numerous claims about the safety of their seeds and GM products. For example, the DDT pesticide was put on the market after being assessed and approved for safety by Monsanto. This chemical is now known to cause cancers, trigger autoimmune diseases and reduce the quality and length of life of millions of people. In my opinion, the manufacturer of a product that requires study should not be allowed to carry out such a study.

"The Case for a GM-free Sustainable World"

The members of the Independent Science Panel of the Institute of Science in Society have reviewed and analyzed numerous scientific evidence and research regarding genetically modified organisms. Many members of the panel signed an "Open Letter from World Scientists to All Governments" in 1999. This letter called for an end to genetically modified organisms; patents on living processes, organisms and more; and a public inquiry regarding food security and the future of agriculture and GMOs.

The following is a summary of their findings.

Have GM crops delivered promised benefits?

GM crops have failed in a few ways to deliver the benefits they have been engineered to deliver. GM crops have cost the U.S. approximately $12 billion worth of lost sales and product recalls as a result of transgenic contamination. In India, for instance, the Bt pesticide failed to be insect resistant up to 100%. This failed resistance phenomenon may result in increased, albeit ineffective, use of additional pesticide, overpopulation of insects and lost crop yields. Bt pesticide failure has also occurred in the U.S., resulting in the same implications.

Major crop failures have occurred as a result of the instability of transgenic lines. Many farmers growing GM crops have reported some level of inaction in their GM crops. The use of Bt in GM plants may also prove to be ineffective as it threatens to create Bt resistant insects and superweeds.

It is difficult to effectively analyze the difference in benefits between genetically modified crops and their conventional counterparts largely due to transgenic contamination. The Bt pesticide used in GM corn has been found in crops grown in remote areas of Mexico and Canada because of wind pollination. It is virtually impossible to grow

GM and non-GM crops separately as cross contamination has become increasingly unavoidable.

Are GM crops unsafe?

GM crops have never been proven "safe." Current safety assessments of GM crops revolve around substantial equivalence, or the comparison of a GMO to its non-GM counterpart. Substantial equivalence as a test is intended to be vague so that companies can readily use the term "substantially equivalent" when referring to their products.

Is the transgenic process itself dangerous?

The only systematic investigation of GMO in the world showed that young rats had "growth-like factor" effects in their stomachs and small intestines. These effects could not be attributed solely to the GM product and were therefore attributed to the transgenic process. Bt proteins used in approximately 25% of genetically modified crops have been found to harm many non-target insects. Some Bt proteins have also been found to cause allergies in humans. In food crops used largely to produce medicines and pharmaceuticals, Bt proteins in the foods could suppress the immune system, create toxicity in the central nervous system and cause various psychological problems.

What does the HIV-1 virus have to do with GM maize?

Incorporated into GM maize is the glycoprotein gene gp120 of the AIDS virus HIV-1. This gene is used in GM corn as an edible vaccine. However, the use of this gene could be detrimental to consumers as the gene can interfere with the immune system, combine with viruses and bacteria and create new pathogens in the body.

How are broad-spectrum herbicides potentially toxic to humans and other species?

Both glufosinate and glyphosate, used in herbicide-tolerant crops, are metabolic poisons that can cause many harmful effects in humans. Glufosinate ammonium is linked to toxicity in the brain, blood, respiratory system and gastrointestinal system. It is also known to cause birth defects in humans and animals, to inhibit beneficial nitrogen-fixing bacteria in the soil, and to be toxic to many beneficial insects.

Glyphosate is also a poison known to disrupt many bodily functions. Exposure to glyphosate in the UK nearly doubled the risk of late abortion, and children born to people who consumed glyphosate had neurobehavioral problems. Glyphosate also caused delayed development of the fetal skeleton in lab rats. Earthworms exposed to the toxin in fields experienced at least 50% mortality and significant intestinal damage in worms that survived.

Can genetic engineering create super-viruses?

One of the most extreme dangers of genetic engineering is the probability of horizontal gene transfer and recombination. Recombination can create viruses and bacteria and cause disease epidemics. For example, in 2001 a genetic engineering experiment unintentionally created a killer mouse virus. By merely recombining genes, it is possible to create viruses that have never before existed. Though the process of recombining genes is currently used for the creation of GM products, it is possible that diseases causing viruses created by recombination could be used as bio-weapons in the future.

Is sustainable agriculture a myth?

Sustainable agriculture is not a myth. Many long-term studies have shown how beneficial sustainable agriculture can be, even in industrialized countries. The use of sustainable agriculture practices can lead to better soil, as these practices reduce soil erosion and increase the water-holding capacity of soil to avert drought. In organic soils, more biological activities can thrive. Insects such as earthworms and other microorganisms are beneficial for the soil as they recycle nutrients and suppress disease.

Sustainable agriculture also allows for a cleaner environment. Unlike genetically modified organisms, no chemicals are put in plants in sustainable farming. Fewer nitrates and phosphates are leached in sustainable agriculture, which leads to less pollution from surface runoff. Fewer pesticides are used in organic farming, and studies have shown no decrease in crop yields because of the decreased use of pesticides. It is also possible to control pests without pesticides, with less of an impact on the surrounding environment and human health, as evidenced by the success of the organic farming industry.

Sustainable agriculture supports biodiversity as opposed to the monocultures found in crops of genetically modified organisms. Because of increased biodiversity, thousands of rice farmers in China have nearly eliminated devastating diseases by using mixed planting techniques in their crops without adding chemicals.

A study performed throughout Europe has shown that organic farming performs better than conventional farming and leads to more favorable conditions in the environment. Organic farming practices use energy efficiently and reduce the amount of carbon emissions in the atmosphere. Sustainable agriculture increases carbon sequestration below the ground by restoring and recycling organic matter in the soil. Sustainable practices are also profitable. Data has shown that when price premiums are factored in, organic systems are more profitable than other systems.

Organic food is better quality and is better for human health. Organic production bans artificial food additives, which have been shown to cause health problems such as heart disease, migraines and hyperactivity.

Are GM crops needed or wanted by the agricultural industry and the rest of the world?

GM crops are neither wanted nor needed by the world for many reasons:

- Widespread hunger is caused by poverty and inequality, not by insufficient food production. A 2005 ActionAid report stated that the increased use of GM crops is contributing to widespread world hunger rather than helping it.
- GM crops increase food insecurity, which leads to more hungry people.
- GM crops also fail to deliver many of the claimed benefits. For example, GM soy yields have decreased significantly, between 5 and 10%.

- GM crops have not reduced the need for herbicides and pesticides to the extent that Monsanto claims. In 2000, the USDA suggested that the average acre of Roundup® Ready corn required 30% more herbicide than conventional corn.
- The cost of GM seed is much more expensive than non-GM seed.
- Due to the lack of research, many consumers and farmers are concerned about the safety hazards that come with genetic modification.

The majority of countries do not endorse the use of GM crops. The reason for the dramatic increase in acreage of GM crops is due to the four major countries that endorse GM products: the United States, Canada, Argentina and China. Countries such as Zambia have refused GM products, and in the Philippines there have been hunger strikes protesting Monsanto's Bt maize. Scientists in Russia are calling for a 10-year ban on GMOs because they say research has proven the foods are dangerous. Other countries have already taken action to remove Monsanto's GMO crops as well. So why hasn't the U.S. followed suit? Could it be that our scientific community is blinded by financial interests?

There has also been much corruption inside Monsanto and the genetic modification industry. Monsanto is a high-risk company, due to the substantial controversy regarding genetically modified products. In April 2003, Innovest Strategic Value Advisors rated Monsanto as having the lowest potential for profitability to investors.

Is there evidence of transgenic instability?
The few examples of plants reported to show stable gene expression have proven to be the exception to the rule, as the majority of transgene plants experience some level of inaction. Many cases of transgene inactivation are never even reported. Even in cases where there is claimed transgenic stability, researchers have found instability. Gene silencing, a major cause of transgenic instability, is the process by which foreign genes integrated into the genome are inactivated so they are no longer expressed. This process is known to be an important part of an organism's defense system against infection.

A second cause of transgenic instability has to do with the transgene's unstable structure. Transgenes have a tendency to break along weak joints and recombine in an incorrect manner with other DNA. This recombination can be potentially dangerous. Investigations have also shown that transgenic instability can arise in later generations.

Can cancer result from GMOs?

Cancer has been shown in many investigations to result from the consumption of GMOs. The report states, "It is now accepted that transgene locus number estimations based on phenotypic segregation ratios are inaccurate due to perturbations of transgene expression via transgene silencing or rearrangement of transgene loci." Evidence shows that transgenic DNA often gets into regions of the genes (our genetic material) that make the DNA prone to doubled stranded breaks. These breaks increase the potential for inactivation of the transgenic DNA and increase the structural instability of the transgene. Said another way, with increased breaks comes increased cancer risk...plain and simple!

Are there Bt resistant crops?

Bt crops are experiencing problems due to target insects developing resistance to Bt. The problem is so large that resistance management strategies have been adopted in the U.S. Farmers have gone so far as to replant non-Bt crops followed by planting largely expressive and toxic Bt crops in an effort to prevent resistance. However, this strategy has been unsuccessful. Even the introduction of multiple toxins into Bt crops has been unsuccessful, as target insects have become resistant to multiple toxins.

Is there evidence for resistant crops?

Much concern exists regarding the possibility of resistant crops to GM chemicals. Resistance is largely due to extensive cross contamination between GM and non-GM crops. A report published in 2001 by Ignacio Chapela and David Quist presented evidence that GM chemicals were found in non-GM corn in Mexico. Wind pollination of Bt corn in the United States and other countries has imposed GM corn on countries that do not endorse it. In Mexico, 95% of the sites sampled were contaminated on average from 10-15%.

The substantial losses for investors in Monsanto and other biotech companies that could result from transgenic cross contamination could potentially bankrupt those companies. Tests performed on the flow of pollen reported that wheat pollen stays airborne for at least one hour, during which time it can be carried over large distances. Farmers growing organic crops have begun legal battles against Monsanto for the contamination of their organic crops.

What flaws are found in the FAO/WHO "Biotechnology and Food Safety" report?
This report was flawed for many reasons. The report:

- claimed many benefits of the technology that were untrue or not proven;
- failed to address some main aspects of food safety such as the use of crops to produce industrial chemicals and medicines and issues concerning the labeling of transgenic foods;
- excluded known hazards such as the toxicity of herbicides from the list of safety concerns;
- made false claims, stating that genetic engineering is no different than conventional agriculture;
- used the "principle of substantial equivalence" to assess risk in genetically modified foods, although the principle is known to be unscientific;
- failed to state long-term impacts of genetically modified foods; and
- ignored scientific studies that have proven the hazards of consuming genetically modified foods.

What is "substantial equivalence" and what are its fallacies?
"Substantial equivalence" refers to the concept that if a new food, such as a GMO, is substantially equivalent in structure and chemical composition to an older food, then the two foods can be treated as though they are equivalent in safety to consumers. The principle is poorly defined and open to much interpretation, however, and for that reason many scientists do not believe substantial equivalence to be useful in deciding upon food

safety. Companies can claim substantial equivalence based on the most expeditious claim. Under this principle, companies can avoid detailed molecular characterization of the GMO, gene expression profiles and other information that would reveal effects that were unintended.

Contrary to what many companies claim, GMOs have never passed any "required" safety tests. The FDA decided in 1992 that safety assessments for genetic engineering are unnecessary, and now safety tests for all GMOs are voluntary. There have been very few independent studies dedicated to the safety of genetically modified foods.

Have some of the studies regarding GM safety been flawed? How?
Few studies regarding the safety of GMOs have been done, and those that have been published are not usually up to high scientific standards. Two reports made before 1999 revealed the harmful effects of GMOs on animals. In one study, several rats fed GM tomatoes developed ulcers on the lining of their stomachs. In humans, life-threatening hemorrhages can result from such ulcers. A second study showed that when mice were fed raw GM potatoes, they developed proliferative growths in the lower small intestine.

A study performed by Dr. Arpad Pusztai and his coworkers revealed that two transgenic lines of GM potatoes were resistant to aphids, and therefore were not substantially equivalent in composition to conventional potatoes. Though many attacked Pusztai's findings, they have yet to be disproved.

What are more transgenic hazards?
Transgenic crops, specifically those containing the Bt toxin, have been found harmful to humans, mice and other animals, and butterflies and other insects, such as those in the Order of Coleoptera, which includes beetles, weevils, stylopids and others. Bt plants negatively impact soil ecology and the fertility of the soil. Crops containing Bt may also be potential allergens for humans.

An experiment found that a Bt strain caused severe human necrosis that killed mice within eight hours from clinical toxic-shock syndrome. Mice fed GM potatoes had a damaged small intestine as well as abnormal mitochondria and degenerated microvilli. Human diseases can also result from chemicals in GM products. Many genes introduced into GM products are from bacteria, which can pose additional risks to humans.

What are suicide seeds and terminator crops?
Terminator crops are genetically engineered crops that contain a "suicide" gene for sterility for male and female seeds. Terminator crops have been field tested in the United States, Europe and Canada. Though there have been large protests against terminator crops, several have been released in North America.

The GM rapeseeds are genetically engineered to be male sterile and are therefore considered terminator crops. The male sterile line of the crop contains a single copy of the "suicide" gene. Crossing the male sterile line with the male restorer line produces an F1 hybrid. By crossing the two lines, anther development can be restored to the plant to produce pollen. The F1 hybrid produced spreads two genes, one for male sterility and one for herbicide tolerance.

How do glufosinate ammonium and glyphosate work and what are some potential dangers?
Glufosinate ammonium is a chemical linked to blood, brain, respiratory and gastrointestinal toxicities. It can also cause birth defects in both humans and mammals. The human brain is sensitive to ammonia and its toxic effects, and the removal of ammonium in the body depends on how it incorporates into glutamate. A large disturbance to glutamate's metabolism could cause a profound impact on health. The effects of the toxin could also have detrimental effects on agriculture. Some pathogens in plants are highly resistant to glufosinate ammonium, while others suffer very negative effects from it.

Glyphosate is a second major herbicide used in genetically modified crops. Glyphosate kills plants by inhibiting the 5-enolPyruvylshikimate-3-phosphate synthase enzyme, which is critical to synthesize amino acids. For glyphosate to be effective, the plant must be growing and exposed to light. Roundup® Ready crops are formulated to be tolerant to

Monsanto's form of glyphosate. These crops are made with two genes, one that reduces the plant's sensitivity to glyphosate and one that helps the plant break down glyphosate.

Glyphosate is dangerous to humans and animals, having the potential to disrupt enzyme systems in the body that utilize PEP. Glyphosate has caused complaints of poisoning in the UK. Symptoms from the ingestion of glyphosate include balance disorder, reduced cognitive capacity, vertigo, seizures, and impaired vision, taste, hearing and smell. Other symptoms such as twitches, tics and headaches have been reported. A study performed in Ontario showed that exposure to glyphosate doubled the risk of late abortion. Other studies have suggested that glyphosate is toxic in mammals and causes synthesis of steroids in animals. Studies have increasingly shown that glyphosate is threatening to both human and animal health.

What is horizontal gene transfer and how might it be hazardous?
Horizontal gene transfer is the transfer of genetic material into the genome of an organism and can occur between organisms of the same or different species. Genetic engineering uses horizontal gene transfer to insert foreign genes and chemicals into new foods. Genetic engineering itself is dangerous, but horizontal gene transfer is possibly the most dangerous. The media finally caught the attention of this danger when a deadly mouse virus was accidentally created in Australia as a result of horizontal gene transfer. An unlimited number of genes can be recombined in an organism, resulting in altered genes that may provoke adverse health consequences. This can cause a great deal of transgenic instability, which can lead to breaking and recombination in the genome and the creation of new unwanted bacteria and viruses.

Why is transgenic DNA more likely to spread horizontally?
Transgenic DNA is more likely to spread horizontally than natural DNA for many reasons. Transgenic DNA often contains new combinations of genes that have never existed. The DNA created for genetically modified organisms is also created to jump into the genome, which enhances the possibility of horizontal gene transfer. The unnatural structure of

transgenic DNA makes it less stable and more likely to break or recombine. Specific enzymes used to speed up the insertion of foreign viral DNA in a genetically modified organism, such as the enzyme integrase, can also function as an enzyme to catalyze the reverse reaction. The continuous expression of an organism to foreign transgenic genes creates great metabolic stress, which can cause instability of the transgenic DNA. In an experiment carried out by Joy Bergelson and her colleagues, transgenic plants were found to be approximately 30 times more likely to spread the herbicide-tolerant trait to non-genetically modified plants nearby than non-transgenic plants. This experiment proved the enhanced ability of transgenic organisms to experience horizontal gene transfer.

Have any definitive experiments of some potential dangers of GMOs been conducted?
Many definitive experiments regarding transgenic DNA in genetically modified foods have been avoided by biotech companies. If definitive studies were conducted by self-regulating biotech companies and transgenic DNA was proved to cause adverse health effects in humans, the GMO industry as a whole would collapse. In one of the few studies on transgenic DNA, published in 2001, the cells of many tissues were found to have been invaded by transgenic DNA. Many studies have stopped short of clear, conclusive evidence regarding the properties of transgenic DNA. Much is still unknown about the nature of DNA and the potential dangers transgenic DNA can cause for consumers ingesting GMOs.

What are some of the benefits of sustainable agriculture?
Sustainable agriculture has many benefits, including a decreased amount of chemicals. Few pesticides and herbicides are necessary to grow organic crops. Because of this, there is less runoff and leaching into the surrounding ecosystem. In non-organic farming, approximately 430 synthetic pesticides are used routinely. The chemicals used are complex and don't degrade easily in the environment. Research on tomato production in California has proven that pesticides are not necessary to protect crops from insects. On organic farms, natural predators of insects that kill crops are abundant, unlike transgenic fields where there is decreased biodiversity. Agricultural biodiversity is necessary for long-term

crop security. In the 2002 FAO meeting on "Biodiversity and the Ecosystem Approach in Agriculture, Forestry and Fisheries," examples were given of how important biodiversity is for agriculture.

Organic crops have been found to have longer shelf lives and higher production yields. Organic crops also have lower costs and higher profits. Organic apples in particular have been more profitable because of quick investment return and price premiums. Organic crops are much better for the environment, as they pose no risk of water pollution or disease for surrounding organisms. Organic foods also help to fight diseases and cancer. The health benefits of organic crops make a great difference in human and animal health.

Nutritional Supplements

An added level of protection against GMO consumption

If after reading this book you decide to make all reasonable attempts to avoid GMOs, you are still likely to be unwittingly exposed to hidden GM contaminants. How does one protect against them? The answer: nutritional supplements.

The following pages provide a summary of specific nutritional supplements to consider as general health supports. Blood Detective Nutritionals, Inc., my supplement company, provides all of these nutritional supplements and other products. Other supplement companies carry comparable products, and you should do your research to compare them with those I have provided in this book. Bottom line: Consider supplementing your diet with some or all of the nutritional supplements I have reviewed here and others depending on your individual health needs.

How Nutritional Supplements Help the Body Deal With GMOs

Ever increasing numbers of people believe our food supply has been nutritionally compromised and want some "nutritional insurance." Nutritional supplements in the form of vitamins, minerals, enzymes, herbs and other natural compounds have been available for decades to meet consumers' demands. Although I believe it is ideal for people to seek the expert advice of trained nutritional specialists before using nutritional supplements, I know that the supplements available from Blood Detective Nutritionals are safe for most people. Furthermore, I believe the risks of taking nutritional supplements are far outweighed by the potential health problems that may arise from consuming GMOs. The old adage applies: "You are what you eat." More accurately, "You are what you absorb and use from what you eat." In the case of Frankenfoods, your health may be compromised as a consequence of your GMO diet.

Concentrated forms of vitamins, minerals, enzymes and other nutritional supplements can improve our immune system, digestive capacity and overall basic nutrition. They can positively affect our sense of well-being, lower disease risk and extend life. Particularly important are the fundamental ways outlined below in which various nutritional products may help our bodies manage GMO consumption. Having said this, I would prefer the complete elimination from the diet of GMOs as opposed to compensating for their presence (at least, perhaps to some small extent), with nutritional supplements.

Extra Protection

GMO labeling laws are in their infancy and GMO ingredients are found in so many products, even in medications. Some non-GMOs may actually contain GMO elements due to cross-contamination during the manufacturing process. Nutritional supplements provide you with an extra level of protection to safeguard your health so your body can handle the potentially damaging effects of GMOs. Below is my short list of nutritional supplements that you might consider taking. Always get the approval of a qualified nutritional health care provider who can advise you based on knowing your medical and health conditions and needs.

The Big Five Body Categories

1. **Toxicity Protection**
2. **Basic Nutrition**
3. **Immune Regulation**
4. **Hormonal Balance**
5. **Digestive Support**

These five basic body categories each contain several nutritional supplement recommendations that may provide extra health support and protection against the accidental consumption of GMOs. The supplements should be taken as directed on the containers' labels. However, you may need more or less of each of these supplements for optimal health protection. Some of the nutritional supplements below may interfere with medications that you may be taking; consider consulting with your health care provider before adding nutritional supplements to your diet. Generally speaking, the nutritional supplements that I discuss in this section are safe when used as directed.

Toxicity, nutritional deficiencies, immune dysregulation, hormone disruption and digestive problems are the five main categories of health that are affected by GMO consumption, according to some reports and studies. Depending on your current level of health; medications you take; sleep, eating, work and exercise habits; lifestyle; and environmental and other influences, your personal nutrition needs may vary significantly from those outlined here. Keep in mind that although I have separated the nutritional compounds below into categories, the nutrients in each category have health benefits that may span more than one or even all categories. For example, probiotics help improve immune function as well as digestion.

Elsewhere in this book I have described the health-endangering aspects of GMOs, and I have explained some of the fundamental ways certain nutritional supplements work in the body. The following recommendations are not necessarily ideal for each individual, but they should serve as a starting point.

Toxicity Protection

A toxin is a substance that, by definition, can cause harm in the body. Depending upon the toxin itself, various cells, tissues, organs and organ systems can be adversely affected. Toxins are of two basic types: those that are produced within the body (endogenous) and those that are taken into the body from the external environment (exogenous). Most tissues in the body attempt to render toxins harmless through a process called detoxification or detoxication. The liver is considered the major organ of detoxification; the kidneys, lungs, skin and digestive tracts also play a major role in detoxification. The liver has a complex and specialized physiology, allowing it to transform toxins and help rid them from the body.

The nutritional supplements described in this section represent the most basic nutrition required by the liver to gather fat soluble toxins and convert them into water soluble toxins so that they can be eliminated via the kidneys into the urine for elimination from the body; essentially, this is known as detoxification. GMOs may provoke toxicity, and the addition of the nutritional supplements outlined below may help reduce the bio accumulation of toxins within the body by enhancing them, a process known as elimination. Therefore, detoxification and elimination go hand in hand for those wishing to take extra preventative health measures against the potential toxic effects of GMOs.

Health Bugs — Probiotics

Probiotics are healthy forms of bacteria and/or yeast that live in our digestive tract. Probiotics have long been known to help our general digestion, enhance absorption of nutrition, support endogenous production of certain B-vitamins, lower cholesterol and regulate immune function. Probiotics also help control excessive inflammation in the body, improve mood and speed up healing of the intestinal tract. For these and other potential health benefits, I recommend probiotics to all of my patients. Probiotics such as *Lactobacillus acidophilus*, *Lactobacillus bifidus* and several other species of "healthy bugs" commonly are packaged and sold as a combination product available in health food stores or from Blood Detective Nutritionals, Inc.

How to supplement: Take 1-2 probiotics/day with a protein food for best results. Go to: http://bit.ly/1dWyb4W

Liver Function

a. **Milk Thistle,** also known as silymarin, is a group of compounds derived from milk thistle seeds consisting of among others of silibinin, isosilibinin, silicristin, and silidianin. Silibinin has also demonstrated *in vitro* anti-cancer effects against human prostate adenocarcinoma cells, estrogen-dependent and -independent human breast carcinoma cells, human ectocervical carcinoma cells, human colon cancer cells and both small and non-small human lung carcinoma cells. Silymarin is known to help reduce oxidative (degenerative stress) in the liver caused by many types of toxins and from the aging process. The liver has over 500 known functions. Thus, silymarin's hepatoprotective effects are fundamentally important when one is concerned about toxicity of any form.

How to supplement: Take 300-600 mg/day with or without food. Go to: http://bit.ly/KT1gRP

b. **Reduced Glutathione** is a tripeptide, the "tri" indicating it is composed of three important amino acids including glycine, glutamic acid and glutamine. Each of these individual amino acids has many varied and important functions to help hinder GMOs' detrimental health effects. Some of the benefits of reduced glutathione include its potent action as a detoxifier of pesticides and metals and as a tissue reparative antioxidant. Glutathione also protects the liver from damage, boosts immunity and protects the liver cells from degenerative toxins and the inflammatory and potentially compromising effects of GMOs.

How to supplement: Take 250-500 mg/day with or without food. Go to: http://bit.ly/KT1gRP

c. **N-Acetyl Cysteine (NAC)** is one of the most important nutritional compounds that a person can add to their diet to maximize resistance to GMOs. NAC has some of the most potent antioxidant effects of all nutrients. All of the reported harmful effects of GMOs, including nutritional, allergic, hormonal and toxic effects, may be offset by including a small amount of NAC each day. NAC is a biologically active amino acid that increases the body's production of glutathione. NAC is also a powerful immune modulator having antiviral, antibacterial, antiparasitic and antifungal effects. NAC is required for a large number of healing reactions as a sulfur donor and a detoxifier of mercury, arsenic and other toxic elements.

How to supplement: Take 500-1000 mg/day, and for best results, away from food. Go to: http://bit.ly/1d1Gzdj

d. **Antioxidants** are nutritional compounds that include vitamin E, vitamin C, selenium, polyphenols and a large variety of natural substances found in abundance in fruits and vegetables, nuts, grains and seeds. Essentially, antioxidants target oxidant species known as free radicals. Free radicals are substances that, although needed for normal physiological processes, in excess cause tissue damage and disease. The human aging process itself has been called a disease of oxidation and thus antioxidants have developed a reputation as anti-aging substances. There is some truth to this and significant scientific evidence that supports our need for diets rich in antioxidants to avoid premature death and disease. Most cancers, autoimmune diseases and diseases of virtually all organs involve some degree of oxidative stress for which antioxidants could help prevent, treat or avoid many diseases all together. There are other substances found within plants such as fruits and vegetables that are essential for antioxidant functions or to assist the detoxification process. Some of these natural compounds needed for antioxidant protection include, natural plant enzymes, fiber, chlorophyll, vitamins, minerals, flavonoids, omega-3 and 6 fatty acids and other substances.

For GMO toxin protective efforts I would suggest taking a concentrate of fruits and vegetables in the form of a nutritional powder. I recommend to my patients three powdered nutritional products:

- Green Detox - http://bit.ly/19Iep6F
- Reds Protect - http://bit.ly/19IewyW
- Longevity Complete – http://bit.ly/1dTZyZk

How to supplement: Take 1-4 scoops/day, diluted in water to taste, 1-3 times per day of each.

Basic Nutrition

Studies have shown more than 70% of Americans are deficient in one or more nutrients. My personal clinical research suggests that various nutritional deficiencies are far more common. Because my practice focuses on nutritional issues, the tests I administer will measure nutrition levels for every patient, and so I detect more cases of deficiencies. The traditional internist, family practitioner or other types of health professionals typically lack the training and therefore do not measure nutrition levels except in the case of very obvious nutritional deficiencies, which are rare. Thus, nutritional deficiencies often go undetected, resulting in increased morbidity and mortality. There is ample evidence that GMOs promote nutritional deficiencies and a variety of health problems. More than ever it is time to augment your non-GMO diet with smart nutritional supplement choices. For most people, I believe that nutritional supplementation is a necessary step, even with the most healthy non-GMO diet, to maximize health potential.

a. **Multivitamin-Mineral combination.** As a first action item to correct the problem, choose a comprehensive multivitamin and mineral formula with the active form of folic acid known as L-5-methyltetrahydrofolic acid (not just "folic acid"). Taking a few multivitamins every day can extend the average lifespan of some individuals and can close the gap between our SAD (Standard American Diet) food choices and quality. Allergies, nutritional deficiencies, toxicity, immune dysregulation and other problems believed to be associated with GMO consumption will undoubtedly require individuals to supplement with a multivitamin *at the very least* as baseline nutritional protection. **How to supplement:** Take 4-6 multivitamin-mineral supplements in 2-3 equally divided dosages/day with or without foods. Go to: http://bit.ly/JumsgT

b. **Vitamin C** depletion in our food supply has been documented and is a major health issue. Vitamin C is required for over 3,000 enzyme reactions that drive tissue repair, detoxification pathways and many other essential reactions in the body. Supplementing one's diet with vitamin C has become essential for helping to offset nutritional depletion resulting from over-farming, acid rain, chemical exposure in the form of pesticides and GMOs.

How to supplement: Take 500 mg, 2-3x/day with or without foods. Go to: http://bit.ly/1aos4j6

c. **Vitamin D3** (cholecalcipherol) is now recognized as one of the most important, if not *the* most important, single nutritional factor directly related to quality and length of life. Studies have determined that the higher one's blood level of vitamin D3, the lower one's risk of dying of anything — and the longer the average life span. Vitamin D3 should be added as a nutritional supplement to offset the toxic, intestinal, neurologic, intestinal and other potential adverse effects of GMO consumption.

How to supplement: Take vitamin D3 based on your blood testing so that your vitamin D3 (25-dihydroxy vitamin D3) is ideally 75 mg/mL. The amount of vitamin D3 in foods and nutritional supplements will not always reach this level. On average, my patients tend to require between 5,000-10,000 IUs of vitamin D3/day. Take vitamin D3 with foods, preferably with healthy fats such as avocados, fish and raw nuts or seeds for better absorption. Go to: http://bit.ly/1dpnNjY

d. **Amino acids** are the building blocks of proteins. Meats, fish, poultry, nuts and seeds all contain proteins. Stress, exercise, certain medications, illness and other factors may increase one's dietary requirements for various amino acids. There are several different classes of amino acids, including essential, non-essential and conditionally essential amino acids. Amino acids are required for tissue repair, immunity and detoxification among many other important physiologic functions throughout the body. The addition of a comprehensive amino acids supplement can improve overall health and wellbeing, including the detoxification process. The amino acid product that I recommend is called Amino Acid Complex.

How to supplement: 2-4 capsules/day. Go to: http://bit.ly/1fdbcBa

Immune Regulation

Preliminary studies on the effects of GMO consumption on the immune system show immune compromise resulting in many varied symptoms. Earlier chapters of this book summarized several studies that outline many of the apparent effects of GMOs on the immune system. The immune system is not only responsible for protecting our body from infections, it also plays an essential role in inflammation control and tissue repair. Several key nutritional supplements have been studied extensively and should be a part of everyone's strategy to help manage the adverse effects of GMOs on immune function.

Most of us are aware of the immune system's essential role in preventing and fighting various infections like the common cold (rhinovirus) and bacterial and fungal infections, but our immune system has other functions vital to helping our bodies manage GMO insults.

The immune system's recognition of substances it considers foreign is essential so that "immune soldiers" can be directed towards "the invaders" to render them harmless or nearly harmless, or to completely destroy them. In fact, humans have several immune systems, but for convenience we group them as "the immune system." White blood cells of various types, including neutrophils, basophils, eosinophils and monocytes, form parts of the cell-mediated immune system. Another part of the immune system, called the humoral immunity, relies on several types of immunoglobulins called IgE, IgA, IgM and IgG. Many of us who believe GMOs are not safe worry that our immune systems may be damaged by them.

Nutritional meal and supplement plans can be designed to provide some measure of support for our immune systems. The selection of nutrients listed below has been proven in scientific studies to positively impact our immunity. However, no studies to date have been performed using any nutritional supplements to combat the potential damaging health effects of GMOs.

Below are summarized a few of my top choices for immune-supportive nutritionals.

a. **Reduced glutathione** is an important immune modulator, meaning it helps to manage both low immune function and hyper-immunity (autoimmune disease). Known as a tripeptide, it is composed of three amino acids: glycine, glutamic acid and cysteine. Each of these amino acids has an important function in the body, but together in the form of reduced glutathione, they help reduce mucous accumulation in the body, protect against toxic oxidizers that destroy and irritate cells in the body, detoxify certain chemicals and perform other important biological functions.
How to supplement: Take reduced glutathione in tablet or capsule form 1-2x/day, 200-400 mg total. Go to: http://bit.ly/KT1gRP

b. **Zinc picolinate** has long been known to be the most biologically friendly or best used form of zinc in the body. Zinc is required for over 175 essential enzyme reactions involved in immune health, tissue repair, detoxification and nervous system function.
How to supplement: Take zinc in the picolinate form 1-2x/day, 25-50 mg/day. Go to: http://bit.ly/1l8hhnN

c. **Immune formula combinations** that contain varied herbal immune modulators provide well-rounded support. My favorite immune herbals include: pomegranate, Indian rhubarb, burdock powder, sheep sorrel powder, slippery elm powder, grapeseed extract, mushroom complex (a mix of Shitake, Reishi and Maiktake mushrooms), arabinogalactan and olive leaf extract.
How to supplement: Take as directed on the label. Go to: http://bit.ly/1elxtJg

d. **Omega-3 fatty acids** are among the most important nutritional products that one can add to a healthy diet. Omega-3 fatty acids are required for hormone balance, immune regulation, cardiovascular protection, and as an antioxidant, anti-inflammatory and tissue reparative agent. These are just a few of the beneficial effects of supplementary omega-3 fatty acids. There is virtually not a cell, tissue, organ or organ system that would not benefit from supplementary omega-3 fats.

e. **How to supplement:** Take between 2-6 grams (2000-6000 mg)/day of a reliable form of omega-3 fatty acid, including those from a fish source or flaxseed oil. Go to: http://bit.ly/1fk3pzH

Hormonal Balance

Everything you eat causes hormonal changes. Foods and certain nutritional compounds can help or hurt your hormonal levels. During the body's natural detoxification processes, potentially detrimental molecules such as hormone metabolites, alcohol, drugs and air pollutants are removed from the blood stream via the liver. Healthy hormone detoxification is a crucial part of the normal functioning of the immune system.

a. **Diindolylmethane (DIM)**, a compound derivative of indole-3-carbinol (I-3-C), is used in the prevention of breast and uterine cancer and may have application in the prevention of an enlarged prostate. Functioning as an antioxidant and phytonutrient, DIM has been identified for its free radical scavenging properties and its ability to improve hormone metabolism in both men and women. A compound derivative of the cruciferous *Brassicaceae* family (e.g., broccoli, cabbage and Brussels sprouts), DIM has estrogen modulation potential (i.e., the altering of estrogen metabolism to 2-hydroxyestrone, "the good estrogen").
    How to supplement: Take 125-250 mg/day with or without food. Go to:
    http://bit.ly/19Iep6F

b. **Vitamin D3** is a pro-hormone now known to be an essential compound for the health and vitality of virtually all cells, tissues and organs. Sunlight exposure will almost never be effective enough to maintain vitamin D3 blood levels of 75 mg/dL to maximally lower overall morbidity and mortality. Therefore, it is recommended that every person add a vitamin D3 supplement to the diet. Vitamin D3 may offset GMO consumption by helping to maintain proper cellular repair, immunity, hormonal balance and lessened inflammation.
    How to supplement: Take vitamin D3 (cholecalcipherol) based on your blood testing so that your vitamin D3 (25-dihydroxy vitamin D3) is at an ideal 75 mg/mL. The amount of vitamin D3 in foods and nutritional supplements will not always reach this

ideal level. On average, my patients tend to require between 5,000-10,000 IUs of vitamin D3 per day. Take vitamin D3 with foods, preferably with healthy fats such as avocados, fish and raw nuts or seeds for better absorption. Go to: http://bit.ly/1dpnNjY

Digestive Supports

Each digestive support indicated below provides important and complementary natural compounds that the body needs to handle toxic insults, such as GMOs, that necessarily must pass through the digestive tract.

Our stomach and small intestine, with the help of pancreatic digestive juices that are secreted into our small intestine, allow us to break down the foods we eat and to extract the vital nutrition for all cellular, tissue and organ system functions. The small intestine is responsible for the absorption of nutrition. Also, the small intestine houses approximately 70% of our immune system. When we consume foods that contain various toxic substances (e.g., GMOs), the small intestine uses its inherent immune system and digestive juices to attempt to break down toxins into harmless substances that can be eliminated from the body. Although the small intestine does not act alone in its efforts to prevent toxins from causing us harm, its vital functions are unique.

The stomach, liver, kidneys and lymphatic organs as well as other organs all work in concert to identify, digest, detoxify and eliminate tens of thousands of toxins, or substances in our foods and environment that can become toxins. GMOs must be digested just like all other foods, and I believe that "supercharging" our digestive and immune ability may go a long way toward enhancing the body's tolerance to GMOs. The digestive enzymes secreted by the pancreas directly into the small intestine are signaled immediately by the foods we eat. Adequate digestion of these foods can reduce allergic tendencies.

GMOs have been shown to provoke allergic reactions in some people. Our pancreatic-small intestine digestion of foodstuffs is not always adequate. My 23 years of clinical nutrition practice has taught me that almost everyone can benefit by adding digestive enzymes with each meal. Taking just a few enzyme supplements can reduce the load on our already taxed pancreas, thus allowing it to regenerate, while simultaneously helping to digest foods. Pancreatic supplements may be derived from animal and/or plant sources. I recommend to my patients a combination of plant and animal enzymes be used because they simply work better together in aiding our digestive efforts than either type does alone.

Fundamentally, the job of enzymes in the body is to aid in the digestive process, reduce inflammation and enhance our immune function. The digestive function is initially the most important in the process of breaking down as completely as possible all components of our foods. The GMO-allergy connection is thought to arise from certain foreign proteins being produced as a direct result of the genetic manipulation of GMOs.

Proteins are composed of varying chain lengths of individual amino acids. GMO abnormal proteins, or proteins that may cause an adverse immune reaction such as an allergy, cause health problems because their protein sequences are deemed unfriendly to our immune system, particularly the portion residing in the small intestine. Digestive enzymes aid in breaking down (digesting) the protein chains of allergic proteins so that they are smaller chains or individual amino acids. The more efficiently the body can digest proteins, with or without the aid of enzyme supplements, the less allergic potential the protein has. However, if a person has an allergy they should not expect that their allergy to a particular protein would resolve or necessarily lessen with improvements with digestion.

a. **Probiotics** are commonly known as healthy bacteria. There are a great number of intestinal microflora in our intestinal tracts that are well known to the body and helpful to the digestive system. Our intestinal flora produce certain B vitamins that our bodies require for energy and to run a large number of enzyme functions that help maintain general health and wellbeing. Probiotics are also known to reduce inflammation in the intestinal tract and to ward off cancer of the intestinal tract by helping the enterocytes (cells of the gut) proliferate normally. Probiotics are essential for managing intestinal digestion, and for maintaining the acid-base balance (known as pH balance) and a normal transit time (the time it takes for fecal matter to move through our intestines towards elimination). The digestive and detoxifying potential of probiotics may help to denature, detoxify or inactivate GMO toxins and other harmful GMO components. **How to Supplement:** Take 1-2 capsules or tablets or use a powdered form of probiotic/day with a meal containing protein. Go to: http://bit.ly/1dWyb4W

b. **Digestive enzymes** refer to the enzymes normally produced by our pancreas, but they can also be supplemented in the form of capsules, tablets, powders and liquids. Enzymes are fundamental for the proper digestion of proteins, carbohydrates and fats. Enzyme supplementation may help the body more fully digest allergic, toxic and other harmful products that may be contained in GMOs. The immune modulating and anti-inflammatory effects of digestive enzymes lend added potential for combating GMOs' negative effects.

How to Supplement: Take 2 or more digestive enzymes as needed with each main meal of the day for a total of 6 or more enzyme supplements/day. Do not take enzymes if you have a history of ulcers. Take your enzymes with your meal either just before or during eating. Go to: http://bit.ly/1fddmB0

c. **Hydrochloric acid (HCL).** Stomach acid is the digestive juice produced by our stomach lining in response to the consumption of protein. Proteins are broken down by hydrochloric acid (HCL) and other digestive components including pepsin. Healthy HCL levels in the stomach, produced in response to the consumption of GMOs, will help the initial digestive process. The stomach is considered the first line of immune defense; the digestive stomach juices are designed to digest organisms in foods and to denature or inactivate certain toxins such as pesticides found in abundance in our food chain. HCL is required for the activation and absorption of calcium into ionized calcium, zinc utilization, magnesium and vitamin B12 absorption.

How to Supplement: Take 1-2 at the beginning of each meal, up to 2x/day or as directed by your health care provider. Do not take this supplement if you have a history of stomach or intestinal ulcers. Go to: http://bit.ly/1elyOzN

d. **Fibers, both soluble and insoluble,** are major structural and nutritional components of fruits, vegetables, grains, beans and legumes. Fibers are considered a form of carbohydrate. The insoluble forms of fiber, such as pectin, aid the overall digestive process and help to remove toxins and waste, including those produced from the digestion of GMOs, from the body via the stool. Soluble fibers such as wheat bran, vegetables and whole grains add bulk to the stool, which helps move foodstuffs more quickly through the stomach and small intestine. Fibers help balance hormones, aid in the ongoing cellular repair necessary to maintain efficient digestive function, and bind to toxins.

How to Supplement: Take 2-4 capsules 2-3x/day with meals. Powdered forms of fiber supplements are available and should be taken as directed. Go to: http://bit.ly/1elyOzN

e. **Glutamine** is an amino acid that is required for tissue repair throughout the body. In fact, glutamine is the most abundant amino acid in the body when requirements are increased under physical stress. To produce lean body tissue including muscle, the body uses glutamine. The more lean organ mass we have, the healthier we generally are and the longer we may live. Glutamine is the major fuel for intestinal cell repair and helps detoxify the body. As an aid to improve immunity, glutamine also helps balance the body's delicate acid-base (pH) balance required for normal physiological reactions to take place. Both physical and toxic traumas increase the body's need for glutamine, which is the potential it holds for helping manage GMO physiologic stressors.

How to Supplement: Take between 1-2 grams (1000-2000 mg/day) of glutamine more than 30 minutes before or 30 minutes after meals daily. Go to: http://bit.ly/1d1Gzdj

As the information in this book shows, there is much we can do to help protect our health from GMOs and other sources of GMO exposure. Our health is ours to safeguard especially when the GMO seed manufacturers place their financial interests ahead of our health. I hope the nutritional guidelines, along with the suggestions and strategies outlined in *Frankenfoods — Controversy, Lies & Your Health*, will help you, your friends and your family to live long, healthy lives.

Note: Dr. Michael Wald owns and operates the nutritional and computer software technology company, Blood Logic, Inc. His company produces dozens of nutritional supplement products and is the exclusive developer and distributor of the Blood Detective™ software programs designed to help health care providers interpret complex laboratory results for their nutritional and other health implications. Dr. Wald acknowledges that nutritional supplements may contain GMO products.

The GMO-free Gluten-free Weight Loss Solution

This book has carefully outlined the potential dangers of GMOs in both the short- and long-term. It is one thing to know which foods are GMO and not eat them, but quite another to live in a world where GMOs are everywhere, obscuring our food choices.

Making the smart food choice to not consume GMOs will help prevent both acute and chronic health problems, including diabetes, intestinal issues and cancers. Not purchasing GMOs will also send an important message to the GMO seed manufacturers such as Monsanto that the public does not want to unwittingly consume foods as part of an uncontrolled scientific experiment.

Gluten, like GMOs, poses additional health risks, making it necessary for me to write a book with the very first GMO-free gluten-free recipes and food plan. This new book, preliminarily titled *The GMO-free Gluten-free Weight Loss Solution*, will be available in 2014. The information in that book has shown amazing potential for helping to manage many difficult health problems and promises to reduce one's risk of premature death by providing practical and healthful recipes over a 40-day period. Just follow the meal plan and eat your way to optimal health! I've provided a 10-day meal plan and sample recipes below as examples of the foods you'll enjoy.

Sample Food Plan and Recipes

Day 1
Breakfast:	Poached Eggs over Steam Sauté Baby Spinach
Lunch:	Fresh Vegetable Soup & Quartered Artichokes
Snack:	Carrot Sticks with Hummus & Roasted Sunflower Seeds
Dinner:	Hearty Chicken Stew & Radicchio-Arugula Salad
Snack:	Sliced Pear

Day 2
Breakfast:	Cinnamon Quinoa with Almond Milk
Lunch:	Black Beluga Bean Lentils with Roasted Rutabaga-Kale Salad
Snack:	Celery Sticks with Guacamole and Roasted Pumpkin Seeds
Dinner:	Lemon-Pepper Baked Halibut, Steam Sauté Swiss Chard & Endive-Beet Salad
Snack:	Sliced Green Apple with Cinnamon

Day 3

Breakfast:	Nonfat Organic Greek Yogurt with Fresh Blueberries
Lunch:	Black Bean Salad with Chopped Cilantro & Fresh Vegetable Soup
Snack:	Celery Sticks with Hummus & Roasted Walnuts
Dinner:	Sesame Mahi Mahi with Steam Sauté Broccoli Florets & Baby Spinach Salad
Snack:	Pink Grapefruit

Day 4

Breakfast:	Gluten-free Steel Cut Oats with Cinnamon Apples
Lunch:	Chickpea Wrap & Avocado-Kale Salad
Snack:	String Beans with Guacamole & Roasted Pecans
Dinner:	Lemon-Chili Roasted Chicken Breast & Arugula-Toasted Almond Salad
Snack:	Naval Orange

Day 5

Breakfast:	Green Super Smoothie with Optional Protein Powder
Lunch:	Petite French Rosemary Lentils & Hearts of Romaine-Toasted Pine Nuts Salad
Snack:	Celery Sticks with Baba Ganoush & Sliced Almonds
Dinner:	Grass Fed Beef Chili and Endive-Beet Salad
Snack:	Sliced Red Apple with Cinnamon

Day 6

Breakfast:	Parsley-Scallion Omelet
Lunch:	Quinoa Taboule Salad & Fresh Vegetable Soup
Snack:	Red Pepper Slices with Hummus & Roasted Pumpkin Seeds
Dinner:	Garlic Wild Rice & Beans over Steam Sauté Swiss Chard & Arugula-Tomato Salad
Snack:	Black Grapes

Day 7

Breakfast:	Nonfat Organic Greek Yogurt with Fresh Strawberries
Lunch:	Chickpea Salad & Fresh Vegetable Soup
Snack:	Zucchini Slices with Guacamole & Roasted Pecans
Dinner:	Grilled Cod with Spaghetti Squash & Finely Chopped Vegetable Salad
Snack:	Sliced Pear

Day 8

Breakfast:	Green Super Smoothie with Optional Protein Powder
Lunch:	Garbanzo Bean Delight & Fresh Vegetable Soup
Snack:	Cucumber Slices with Hummus & Roasted Pumpkin Seeds
Dinner:	Gingered Wild Salmon with Steam Sauté Broccoli Florets & Avocado-Kale Salad
Snack:	Pink Grapefruit

Day 9

Breakfast:	Poached Eggs over Steam Sauté Baby Spinach
Lunch:	Sunflower Wild Rice & Fresh Zucchini Salad
Snack:	Carrot Sticks with Hummus & Sliced Almonds
Dinner:	Turkey Chili with String Beans & Arugula-Radicchio Salad
Snack:	Naval Orange

Day 10

Breakfast:	Gluten-free Steel Cut Oats with Fresh Blueberries
Lunch:	Aduki Bean Wrap & Fresh Vegetable Soup
Snack:	Cherry Tomatoes & Roasted Walnuts
Dinner:	Lemon-Pepper Baked Halibut with Asparagus & Baby Spinach Salad
Snack:	Sliced Green Apple with Cinnamon

Sample Recipes

Parsley-Scallion Omelet

3 fresh organic eggs
1/4 cup organic flat leaf parsley, chopped
1/4 cup organic scallions, chopped
Pinch turmeric and pink salt

Place eggs into medium bowl and whisk for 1 minute. Add remaining ingredients and whisk for a few seconds. Heat 1 tsp. coconut oil in medium size pan and pour in the omelet mixture. Bring to gentle bubbling and carefully fold over to half-moon; cook to a light brown. Serve immediately.

Substitute your favorite vegetables and herbs for more delicious omelet recipes, such as:

Tomato-Basil Omelet:

1/4 cup organic grape or cherry tomatoes, chopped
1/4 cup organic basil leaves, chopped
Pinch cayenne and pink salt

Poached Eggs over Baby Spinach
2 fresh organic eggs
2 cups water
2 tablespoons olive oil
Pinch paprika
Pinch pink salt
Poach 2 eggs and place atop fresh baby spinach. Add the olive oil, paprika and pink salt.
If you do not have an egg poacher, you may do the following:
Bring water to a gentle boil and turn down to a simmer in medium size pot. Crack one egg
into a small bowl or cup and bring very close to heated water, pouring the egg in very
slowly and gently so as not to break the yolk. You may use a spoon to bring the egg white
closer to its egg yolk for appearance. Do the same with the second egg. Turn off heat and
cover to stand for 4 minutes. Remove eggs with a slotted spoon.

Finally, I believe that a GMO-free, gluten-free lifestyle promotes lean body weight,
accelerated metabolism, mental clarity and abundant energy. As a practical suggestion, if
you find the following recipes seem too difficult to incorporate into your lifestyle, my
suggestion is simply this: Become familiar with the GMO-free foods mentioned in this book,
and keep abreast of any new GMOs being introduced into the food market so you can avoid
them.

By consulting and using the extensive health plan and recipes in my upcoming book,
The GMO-free Gluten-free Weight Loss Solution, you will gain a solid working knowledge of
which foods are both gluten-free and GMO-free.

Hippocrates said, "Let food be thy medicine and let medicine be thy food." Few words
ever uttered are as true as these. Be mindful of his words — eat well and enjoy life.

REFERENCES

"65 Health Risks of GM Foods." Institute for Responsible Technology. http://responsible
technology.org/gmo-dangers/65-health-risks/2notes.

Antoniou, M., Robinson, C., and Fagan, J. "GMO Myths and Truths Version 1.3b." *Earth Open
Source* (last modified June 2012). http://earthopensource.org/files/pdfs/GMO_Myths_and_
Truths/GMO_Myths_and_Truths_1.3b.pdf.

Bessin, R. "Bt-Corn: What It Is and How It Works." *College of Agriculture, Food and Environment.*
University of Kentucky, 2004. http://www2.ca.uky.edu/entomology/entfacts/ef130.asp.

Bonham, K. "Allergic to Science–Proteins and Allergens in Our Genetically Engineered Food."
Scientific American Blogs (blog), May 39, 2013. http://blogs.scientificamerican.com/guest-blog/
2013/05/30/allergic-to-science-proteins-and-allergens-in-our-genetically-engineered-food/.

Butcher, M. "Genetically Modified Food - GM Foods List and Information." *Disabled World*,
September 22, 2009 (last modified June 28, 2013). http://www.disabled-world.com/fitness/
gm-foods.php.

Byrne, P. "Labeling of Genetically Engineered Foods," Fact Sheet No. 9.371. Colorado State
University Extension, 2010. http://www.ext.colostate.edu/pubs/foodnut/09371.html.

Chichosz, G., and Wiackowski, S. "Genetically Modified Food — Great Unknown." *Polski
Merkuriusz Lekarski*, no. 33 (2012): 59-63.

"Commonly Asked Questions About the Food Safety of GMOs." Monsanto. http://www. monsanto.com/newsviews/Pages/food-safety.aspx.

Cranshaw, W. *"Bacillus Thuringiensis"* Fact Sheet No. 5.556. *Insect Programs.* Colorado State University Extension (last modified September 2010). http://www.ext.colostate.edu/pubs/ insect/05556.html.

"DNA GMO Testing of Seed, Grain, Feed and Food." Biogenetic Services, Inc. http://www. biogeneticservices.com/plant_dnagmo.htm.

EFSA Panel Working Group on Animal Feeding Trials. "Safety and Nutritional Assessment of GM Plants and Derived Food and Feed: The Role of Animal Feeding Trials." *Food & Chemical Toxicology.* no. 46. (2008): S2-70.

Ewan, S., and Pusztai, A. "GM Food Debate." *The Lancet.* no. 9191 (1999): 1726-27. http://www. thelancet.com/journals/lancet/article/PIIS0140-6736(05)76708-8/fulltext.

Falco, T. "Bovine Growth Hormone (rBST) and Dairy Trade." American University, 1997. http:// www1.american.edu/TED/bst.htm.

Flynn, L., and Gillard, M. "Pro-GM Food Scientist 'Threatened Editor'." *The Guardian*, October 31, 1999. http://www.guardian.co.uk/science/1999/nov/01/gm.food.

Gallucci, J. "GMOs in Food: Genetically Modified Food & Our Kids ." *Long Island Press* (last modified November 04, 2010). http://archive.longislandpress.com/2010/08/12/gmos-in-food-genetically-modified-food-and-our-kids/.

"Genetically Modified (GM) Foods." *Better Health Channel*. Deakin University, July 2011. http://www.betterhealth.vic.gov.au/bhcv2/bhcarticles.nsf/pages/Genetically_modified_foods.

"Genetically Modified Organisms (GMO); Harmful Effects of the Agent." *School of Public Health*. University of Minnesota, Fall 2003. http://enhs.umn.edu/current/5103/gm/harmful.html.

"Genetic Engineering: Feeding the EU's Livestock." *GMO Compass*, December 07, 2006. http://www.gmo-compass.org/eng/grocery_shopping/processed_foods/153.animal_feed_genetic_engineering.html.

"GM Crops Do Not Increase Yield Potential." Institute for Responsible Technology (last modified December 26, 2011). http://responsibletechnology.org/docs/gm-crops-do-not-increase-yields.pdf.

"GM Nutritionally Enhanced and Altered Crops." GM-Free Cymru (last modified May 14, 2009). http://www.gmfreecymru.org/pivotal_papers/altered_crops.html.

"GMO Risks." *All About GMOs*. GMO Awareness. http://gmo-awareness.com/all-about-gmos/gmo-risks/.

Grannum, G. "Comprehensive List of GMO Products." *Shift Frequency*, October 02, 2012. http://shiftfrequency.com/comprehensive-list-of-gmo-products/.

Hirschler, B., and Kelland, K. "Study on Monsanto GM Corn Concerns Draws Skepticism." *Reuters LONDON* (blog), September 19, 2012. http://www.reuters.com/article/2012/09/19/us-gmcrops-safety- idUSBRE88I0L020120919.

Honeycutt, Z. "Stunning Corn Comparison: GMO versus NON GMO." *MomsAcrossAmerica.com* (blog), March 15, 2013. http://www.momsacrossamerica.com/stunning_corn_comparison_gmo_versus_non_gmo.

Hoppichler, J. "Bt-plants as a Potential Contributing Factor to Colony Collapse Disorder (CCD)" (presentation, Federal Institute for Less-Favoured and Mountainous Areas, Vienna). http://www.gmo-free-regions.org/fileadmin/files/gmo-free-regions/Hoppichler_presentation.pdf.

Independent Science Panel. "The Case for a GM-free Sustainable World." Institute of Science in Society & Third World Network (last modified June 15, 2003). http://www.psrast.org/caseforGMfreeW.pdf.

Kariyawasam, K. "Legal Liability, Intellectual Property and Genetically Modified Crops: Their Impact on World Agriculture." *Pacific Rim Law & Policy Journal*. no. 3 (2010): 459-85. http://digital.law.washington.edu/dspace-law/bitstream/handle/1773.1/511/19PacRimL&PolyJ459 (2010).pdf?sequence=3.

Kumar, S., Chandra, A., and Pandey, K. "Bacillus Thuringiensis (Bt) Transgenic Crop: An Environment Friendly Insect-Pest Management Strategy." *Journal of Environmental Biology*. no. 5 (2008): 641-53.

"Labeling Food and Ingredients Developed from GM Seed." Monsanto (last modified March 2013). http://www.monsanto.com/newsviews/Pages/food-labeling.aspx.

Lendman, S. "Potential Health Hazards of Genetically Engineered Foods." *Global Research*. The Centre for Research on Globalization (last modified October 17, 2013). http://www.globalresearch.ca/potential-health-hazards-of-genetically-engineered-foods/8148.

Managing Global Genetic Resources: The U.S. National Plant Germplasm System. National Academy Press, 1991. http://www.nap.edu/openbook.php?record_id=1583&page=R1.

"'March Against Monsanto' Protesters Rally Against U.S. Seed Giant and GMO Products." *Huffington Post Green*, May 25, 2013. http://www.huffingtonpost.com/2013/05/25/march-against-monsanto-gmo-protest_n_3336627.html.

Mercola, J. "Why Are Toxin Proteins Genetically Engineered Into Your Food?" *Mercola.com* (last modified September 26, 2011). http://articles.mercola.com/sites/articles/archive/2011/09/26/why-are-toxin-proteins-genetically-engineered-into-your-food.aspx.

Mercola, J., and Droege, R. "How Do You Know if Your Food is Genetically Modified?" *Mercola.com*, January 24, 2004. http://articles.mercola.com/sites/articles/archive/2004/01/24/gm-foods.aspx.

Miraglia, M., Berdal, K., and Brera, C. et al. "Detection and Traceability of Genetically Modified Organisms in the Food Production Chain." *Food and Chemical Toxicology*, no. 42 (2004): 1157-80.

"More Than 70 Consumer Groups, Dairies and Environmental Organizations Urge Ohio Governor Strickland Not to Implement Ban on Milk Hormone Labeling." Center for Food Safety (last modified 2008). http://www.centerforfoodsafety.org/issues/303/seeds/press-releases/870/more-than-70-consumer-groups-dairies-and-environmental-organizations-urge-ohio-governor-strickland-not-to-implement-ban-on-milk-hormone-labeling.

Murray, J. "Genetically Modified Animals." *brainwaving.com* (blog), July 28, 2010. http://www.brainwaving.com/2010/07/28/genetically-modified-animals/.

Neuamerica. "Huge List of Genetically Modified Grocery Frankenfoods." *Rumor Mill News* (blog), February 21, 2004. http://www.rumormillnews.com/cgi-bin/archive.cgi?read=44805.

"Nutritionally Enhanced Plants." *Plant Science for a Better World*. Crop Science Society of America. https://www.crops.org/about-crops/nutritionally-enhanced-plants.

"PCR to Detect Genetically Modified Organisms (GMOs) Field Trip." BioPharmaceutical Technology Center Institute. http://www.btci.org/k12/bft/GMOpcr/GMOpcr_background.html.

"Pew Initiative on Food and Biotechnology, Genetically Modified Crops in the United States." Pew Initiative on Food and Biotechnology (last modified August 2004). http:/www.pewtrusts.org/uploadedFiles/wwwpewtrustsorg/Fact_Sheets/Food_and_Biotechnology/PIFB_Genetically_Modified_Crops_Factsheet0804.pdf.

"Process of Developing Genetically Modified (GM) Crops." *African Biosafety Network of Expertise (ABNE)*. The New Partnership for Africa's Development. 2010. http://www.nepadbiosafety.net/subjects/biotechnology/process-of-developing-genetically-modified-gm-crops.

"Recombinant Bovine Growth Hormone." American Cancer Society (last modified February 02, 2011). http://www.cancer.org/cancer/cancercauses/othercarcinogens/athome/recombinant-bovine-growth-hormone.

"Roundup® Ready Crops." *SourceWatch.* Center for Media and Democracy (last modified December 10, 2013). http://www.sourcewatch.org/index.php/Roundup_Ready_Crops.

Sayer, J. "New Study Finds GM Corn and Roundup® Causes Cancer in Rats." *Green MedInfo.com* (blog), September 19, 2012. http://www.greenmedinfo.com/blog/alert-gmo-corn-and-roundup-caused-cancer-and-killed-rats.

Sennebogen, E., and Gallagher, F. "10 Common Genetically Modified Foods." *HowStuff Works.com*, August 2009. http://recipes.howstuffworks.com/5-common-genetically-modified-foods.htm.

Smith, J. "Are Genetically Engineered Foods Promoting Autism?" The Institute for Responsible Technology, 2012. http://www.responsibletechnology.org/autism.

Society of Toxicology Working Group. "The Safety of Genetically Modified Foods Produced Through Biotechnology." *Toxicological Sciences.* no. 1 (2003): 2-8. http://toxsci.oxfordjournals.org/content/71/1/2.full.

Stevenson, H. "GMO Toxins Are in Nearly All Pregnant Women & Fetuses." *Gaia Health* (last modified September 17, 2012). http://gaia-health.com/gaia-blog/2012-09-17/gmo-toxins-are-in-nearly-all-pregnant-women-fetuses/.

"The Food/Feed Safety Assessment." Monsanto. http://www.monsanto.com/newsviews/Documents/food_feed_safety.pdf.

"They Eat What? The Reality of Feed at Animal Factories." *Union of Concerned Scientists.* Center for Science and Democracy (last modified August 08, 2006). http://www.ucsusa.org/ food_and_agriculture/our-failing-food-system/industrial-agriculture/they-eat-what-the-reality-of.html.

Wald, M. "The GMO-free Gluten-free Weight Loss Solution." *Integrated Medicine of Mt. Kisco* (blog), January 26, 2014. http://www.intmedny.com/integrated-medicine-blog/?category=GMO.

Weber, J. "GMO Alert: Startling New Research." *Live in the Now* (last modified May 23, 2012). http://www.liveinthenow.com/article/gmo-alert-startling-new-research-study.

West, M. "Russia Calls for 10-Year Ban on GMOs. Why Hasn't the U.S.?" *Live in the Now* (last modified January 15, 2014). http://www.liveinthenow.com/article/russia-calls-for-10-year-ban-on-gmos-why-hasnt-the-u-s.

Wikipedia contributors. "Bovine Somatotropin." *Wikipedia, The Free Encyclopedia* (last modified January 31, 2014). http://en.wikipedia.org/wiki/Bovine_somatotropin.

Wikipedia contributors. "Detection of Genetically Modified Organisms." *Wikipedia, The Free Encyclopedia* (last modified January 15, 2014). http://en.wikipedia.org/wiki/Detection_of_genetically_modified_organisms.

Wikipedia contributors. "Genetically Modified Food; Highly Processed Derivatives Containing Little to No DNA or Protein." *Wikipedia, The Free Encyclopedia* (last modified January 30, 2014). http://en.wikipedia.org/wiki/Genetically_modified_food#Highly_processed_derivatives_containing_little_to_no_DNA_or_protein.

Wikipedia contributors. "Intellectual property." *Wikipedia, The Free Encyclopedia* (last modified January 29, 2014). http://en.wikipedia.org/wiki/Intellectual_property.

Wikipedia contributors. "Monsanto." *Wikipedia, The Free Encyclopedia* (last modified February 1, 2014). http://en.wikipedia.org/wiki/Monsanto.

Wikipedia contributors. "Staphylococcus Aureus Beta Toxin." *Wikipedia, The Free Encyclopedia* (last modified January 30, 2014). http://en.wikipedia.org/wiki/Staphylococcus_aureus_beta_toxin.

Wilson, R. "Maine Becomes Second State to Require GMO Labels." *The Washington Post GovBeat* (blog), January 10, 2014. http://www.washingtonpost.com/blogs/govbeat/wp/2014/01/10/maine-becomes-second-state-to-require-gmo-labels/.

"Why Do We Want to Spray More Agent Orange on Our Crops? Are We at War with Ourselves (and Our Children)?" Alliance for Natural Health USA, February 07, 2012. http://www.anh-usa.org/agent-orange-on-our-crops/.

Index

ILSI Crop Composition Database 93, 94

immune regulation 112, 119

inflammatory bowel 2, 29, 61, 81

insect 18, 32, 37, 40, 42, 67, 69, 70, 71, 72, 81, 98, 99, 100, 103, 105, 108

insecticide(s) 13, 67, 69, 71, 72, 96

insecticide resistance 96

intellectual property law 62

Lancet 29, 73, 74

Lupus 2, 80

media 15, 17, 74, 75, 76, 107

Monsanto 3, 5, 9, 13, 14, 20, 29, 31, 34, 39, 41, 47, 57, 62, 63, 65, 80, 88, 89, 94, 97, 102, 104, 128

Multiple Sclerosis 2, 80

natural selection 16, 39, 40, 76

organic 2, 23, 56, 58, 59, 60, 64, 100, 101, 104, 108, 109

papayas 41, 59, 83

PCR (polymerase chain reaction) 47, 52, 54

pesticide(s) 11, 12, 16, 18, 26, 32, 35, 36, 39, 42, 43, 49, 54, 59, 61, 66, 67, 71, 77, 78, 96, 97, 98, 100, 101, 102, 108, 114, 118, 126

pesticide factory 11

pig(s) 28, 29, 50, 51, 84

Posilac 86

potatoes 29, 30, 42, 46, 48, 73, 105

pregnant 20, 21, 35, 36

protein(s) 12, 18, 20, 29, 30, 31, 32, 33, 35, 47, 48, 49, 52, 53, 56, 66, 67, 69, 70, 71, 86, 92, 99, 114, 118, 125, 126

puberty 34

Putzsai 48, 49, 74, 105

rats 28, 29, 48, 73, 77, 80, 94, 99, 100, 105

rBGH (recombinant bovine growth hormone) 34, 44

rBST (recombinant bovine somatotropin) 86, 87, 88